Do You Want
What We I
Beat Canc

Active Cancer Therapy Support

Do You Want to Know What We Did to Beat Cancer?

By Robert Olifent

Published by

Active Cancer Therapy Support

Published March 2017
Copyright © 2017

To order further copies of our book, or to find out more about our support facilities, please contact us or visit our website. We provide empowering talks and educational workshop seminars to share our experience of how we wrecked the bodily environment that supports cancer to thrive. Sue and I have a passion to help people through nutritional health and lifestyle coaching.

07976 665781

Website: www.cancer-acts.com

Email: info@cancer-acts.com

www.cancer-acts.com

info@cancer-acts.com

Book Review

By Michael Burt, ND, RGCRN

Qualified at: The British College of Naturopathy.
Registered by: The General Council & Register of Naturopaths.
Founder of Brabant House Clinic, Surrey.

As a qualified naturopath of over 30 years, I utilize various forms of complementary medicine. I am not a medical doctor and I do not practice orthodox medicine.

Cancer, it would appear, can be precipitated by a wide range of causative factors. I found this book to be a fascinating account of a husband and wife's cancer journey. Through pain and grief in the loss of close loved ones with cancer, to being set on a journey of research and discovery.

In my opinion, as a book review, I believe the following is fair comment:-

The book is packed full of useful information, set out in a clear and concise manner. I found the book to be an intriguing account of how Robert Olifent set about devising a dietary and lifestyle regime to help support his wife Sue regain her health. Instead of dying of cancer within a short period of time as had been predicted, Sue is alive and very well six years later. Another interesting thing is that other health problems cleared up too.

The information provided is clearly the result of extensive and painstaking research and an excellent basis for a naturopathic health program.   Since "prevention is better than cure" I would recommend this book to anybody, irrespective of whether they have cancer or not, who might wish to know what pragmatic steps can be taken to help improve, restore and maintain health.

Michael Burt, ND.

Brabant House Clinic,
Contact details on page 160

Quotations

"The doctor of the future will no longer treat the human frame with drugs, but rather will cure and prevent disease with nutrition."

Thomas Edison

"The part can never be well, unless the whole is well."

Plato

"The most deadly weapons used by man in committing suicide are the knife, fork, and spoon."

Dr. R. L. Greene,

"The truth is incontrovertible, malice may attack it, ignorance may deride it, but - at the end - there it is."

Winston Churchill

Contents

Contents

Acknowledgements

Our sincere thanks go to our wonderful friends and family who in various ways have been incredibly supportive in our lives. Some have played an active part in the production of this book and our website. We would like to acknowledge these wonderful people for their encouragement, direction and for standing by us through the storm, bringing positivity and joy into our lives throughout difficult and turbulent times.

Derek Bolton, Christine Stala,

Maverick Bailey, Valerie Bailey,

Christine Scott, Jordan Olifent,

Stella Skidmore, Kristina Jones,

Mark and Heather Day,

Rita, Jody and Stephen Callaghan,

Neil Butterworth, Lynda Markarian

The Legal Bit Out of The Way

It is a sad reality to the state of our blame and claim culture when this sort of legal disclaimer has to be made. The following information contained within this book is for 'information purposes only' and does not constitute specific nutritional or medical advice in individual cases.

The information contained herein is inarguably what we chose to do when my wife was faced with cancer in January 2011. It is hoped that through our experience people will grasp the concepts of what we chose to do and the logic behind what we did. It is strongly recommended that anyone currently going through chronic illness should consult a professional healthcare or nutritional practitioner, just as we did. It is also advised for the reader to do their own research and then to formulate their own personal healthcare strategies based on logical and well balanced information.

Our belief is that information is the 'key' to the vast array of armoury at our disposal when going through serious health issues. However, to open the gates to that armoury you need to put the key in the lock and turn, which means an action on your part! Life in general does not come with guarantees and this is certainly true of conventional cancer treatments as well as naturopathic. We believe it is simply sensible reasoning to base important health decisions on information and with eyes wide open, whichever pathway is chosen.

My heart goes out to those who are in health crises at the moment and I pray that the information contained within these pages may bring comfort, strength and lead to ultimate wellbeing.

Foreword

The basic principle of building up the body and the immune system whilst going through cancer has to be simple common sense, who could really argue with this? To have an understanding of the many well documented issues that serve to 'feed' or 'fight' cancer will give the person who has this knowledge a greater edge over this scourge of western society i.e. 'CANCER'.

Simply making changes to poor nutritional and lifestyle 'habits' could serve to stack the odds in your favour. Would you pour petrol on a bonfire to put it out? Of course not! Then by the same concept we must not provide cancer with the ideal biological/environmental conditions that it needs to thrive. How can you know this, you may ask? By acquiring well documented knowledge and thinking logically 'outside the box'. Plus very importantly by implementing this knowledge and taking personal responsibility. Our heart is to give our story for people to make up their own minds in the health choices available to them. It is also our hope that this knowledge may serve to get people eating healthier and becoming healthier, thereby taking the massive strain off our crumbling National Health Service and lessening unnecessary suffering of humanity.

Through many tears, sorrow and heartache to the positivity of healing through natural nutritional pathways, this is simply 'our experience', from hopelessness to the reversal of cancer. Our passion is to share our experience to help encourage others, with Sue now being cancer free.

If you feel that the information contained within this book may be of benefit to anyone currently going through cancer then we would encourage you to share what you have learned with others.

Introduction

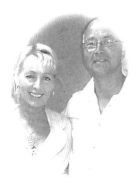

The following information is in remembrance of my father John David Olifent and mother Sheila June Olifent, whom died with cancer in May and June 2008 respectively. Additionally my father in law J. Eamon Callaghan, whom died with cancer in 1991 and my wonderful uncle Tony Harrison too who also died with cancer in 2012. During these traumatic times I witnessed some disturbing and seriously contradictory practices within conventional orthodox cancer treatments and standard of care. I felt extremely uncomfortable with these experiences which prompted me to ask questions and to research the reasons why one person in two, (the flip of a coin) will get cancer in their lifetime, as these are I understand the current statistics from the Cancer Research UK (CRUK).

My studies became fairly extensive and I subsequently amassed a wide ranging and large body of knowledge in traditional medical healthcare, alternative therapies, nutritional books/literature and various CD/DVD teaching/lectures plus I attended various training courses and workshops. The more knowledge I gained, the clearer the picture came to me as to what we in western society are doing to ourselves nutritionally and through our inherited or chosen lifestyles. It became self-evident that we have become a sick nation of heart disease, cancer, diabetes, obesity, psychological disorders, MS, arthritis, dementia, fibromyalgia and other auto immune diseases etc. but this does not have to be so.

Clearly it would be unwise to suggest that there is any single reason for these problems, or for that matter to suggest any single type of snake oil cure, but there are definite reasons for our nation's ills which we have come to more or less accept that this is the way life is as we age. However, having the ability to accept that there may be something fundamentally out of sync in westernised society is the beginning to wisdom and having the ability to make better choices to prevent disease or might I suggest, even to turn things around for total recovery.

I have been involved in researching cancer and health issues since 2008 following my parents passing away. Both my wife and I have a passion to share what we have learned and experienced. As I cannot claim to be a medical professional, nutritionist or qualified naturopath it is advisable that anyone who is thinking about going down the route of nutritional therapy or alternative therapies should consult a professional healthcare or nutritional practitioner in order to ensure that there are no conflicts with any medications or treatments that you may currently be on. I have drawn the following information together from a wide and wonderful body of research that is freely available but, strangely enough, seems to be largely ignored by orthodox cancer society's/charity's and medical establishments, being deemed to be outside the scope of scientific clinical trials and patentable synthetic chemical based pharmaceutical drugs.

The following information is the basis of 'what we did' when my wife was faced with cancer and given no hope by the medical establishment and she is now cancer free.

The information contained herein is what we believe to be a common sense approach, not rocket science. There may well be more to know and it is up to each individual to gain as much knowledge as they can in order to make 'informed decisions' about their own treatment options.

All too often people are rushed and railroaded down a one track fits all sledgehammer to crack a nut system, that cannot or will not look at any other way but chemotherapy, radiotherapy or surgery to treat cancer. I would pose this question: do these conventional cancer treatments deal with any root cause issues as to why the person has been susceptible to cancer in the first place? If your answer is no, then is it not logical that the body is still as vulnerable to spawning cancer as it was in the first instance? Perhaps this is even more so, due to the carcinogenic (cancer causing) cytotoxic nature of orthodox cancer treatments (chemotherapy and radiotherapy) along with the ravenous indiscriminate destruction they have on depleting the body's foundational health, immune system and cells.

To me there seems to be something seriously questionable about cancer standard of care treatments that in order to make you healthy would cause hair, teeth and nails to fall out, to vomit, destroy the immune system, damage sensory organs, cause chemical and radiation burning all with long term debilitating health consequences. Oh, and according to the drug manufacturers own material safety data sheets (MSDS) many cause cancer too!

> "One of the biggest tragedies of human civilization is the precedence of chemicals over nutrition."
>
> Dr Richard Murray

Yes, that shocked me at first, but I do recommend that you research this for yourself!

Our experience is that there are other options to consider that are safe, nontoxic and highly effective in building up the body's immune system. These natural options not only help to create a healthy body but a body in which cancer struggles to thrive. However this requires a degree of knowledge, self-discipline and taking personal responsibility.

Remember, the information contained herein is 'not medical guidance' and we are not giving specific advice, it is simply sharing our personal experience. This is for you to use your own

God given rationale, but please base this rationale on knowledge and hard facts rather than simply blind trust of the person in the white coat.

I believe that it is good practice to put everyone and everything under close scrutiny when it comes to your health. Question everything that is being said to you, including the information contained within the pages of this book, as well as the medical profession.

Ask yourself;

Who is it that is talking?

What are they saying?

Why are they saying it?

What's in it for them?

Are they truly able to speak freely?

Are they qualified to speak about nutrition?

Are they qualified to speak about medication?

Is there bias in what is being said?

Make sure that you understand the principles of any treatment options proposed to you and rationalise them. Weigh up the pros and cons of the medical approach or naturopathic approach and take time to do this. Most likely the cancer has been there from between five to fifteen years so is there really such a massive rush to make such important health decisions?

I think that it is a wise person who bases their actions and decisions on a good balance of knowledge and all options available.

The Bombshell

Having researched and collated a substantial amount of information in the years following my parents passing away, we were devastated to find out in January 2011, my wife Sue had been diagnosed with a large tumour on her liver and three smaller growths on the pancreas.

Sue started to experience painful stabbing sensations in her abdomen whenever she ate, actually when food was first placed in her mouth, even before swallowing. Sue subsequently lost one and a half stone in weight quite rapidly, which in itself was seriously worrying as Sue was slim anyway. Arrangements were made to have scans where it was discovered that she had a 60x 50x 54ml tumour (two and a half inch) on her liver and three suspect nodules on the tail end of her pancreas.

Sue sat with the doctor and was shown the scanned images on the computer monitor screen. The doctor specifically pointed the tumours out explaining the dire location of the tumour on the liver, where it was attached and compressing/strangulating the bile duct tubes which go in and out, "like charring Cross Station" to quote the doctors words.

He told Sue that he was so very sorry; whether the tumour on the liver was benign or malignant the situation was not good due to its critical location. He explained that he had not seen a cancer of this type in a woman of Sue's age and that she should prepare for the worst because it would be inoperable being in such a highly sensitive area. The Doctor then recommended that Sue should take Temazepam sleeping tablets which he was prescribing to her, "Because she was going to need them" were his very words. The Doctors leaving words were: "I am so very sorry". Sue was so distraught by this news, that she went out from the doctors and bought twenty five pounds worth of goodbye cards to send to her family and friends.

In Sues Words, "When I came out of the doctor's office after being told the news I felt numb. I got on a bus into town looking around at all the people chattering away, things seemed surreal. All that kept going around my head was that I have got cancer, cancer, cancer! I felt like screaming on the bus, I have cancer, I'm going to die! Everyone just kept chattering away oblivious to the turmoil going on inside of me.

I went to the card shop and spent an hour choosing special cards for people I love and then went on to collect my prescription for sleeping tablets that my doctor had prescribed to me earlier. That's when my tears just wouldn't stop. No one approached me to ask if I was ok, but I was so glad they didn't.

My tears continued on the bus home as I thought about telling my son, oh my, how on earth do you tell your child something like this, he was only sixteen. I thought my role in life was to see Jordan get a good job, get married and to be a good grandma to his children. This was now being snatched away, how could this be happening to me, I was only forty five?

Then there was my husband Rob, he wasn't well in himself, and was still grieving from losing his parents to cancer two years earlier. I felt that this would break him again. I decided there and then that I was not going to tell them.

I telephoned my best friend Lynda, as I desperately needed someone to talk to. I spent most of the time reassuring her that I would be ok, although inside I didn't believe my own reassuring words. How could I believe that I was going to be ok with the tremendous pain I was having, the weight loss, seeing the tumours on the screen and hearing the words of what my doctor had just explained to me.

I then telephoned Martin my boss, because I couldn't cope with the thought of going into work and breaking down crying in front of customers.

I spent the afternoon writing the cards out to friends and family, but the tears would not stop as I kept looking at the clock waiting for my family to come home. I had to pull myself together as I felt they must not see me like this. Then finally I heard a key in the door, it was Rob.

My heart was racing and I couldn't stop shaking. I could not hide my feelings and emotions from him as I had planned too, it was just impossible. Rob's response was dismay and it seemed that he had difficulty in it registering with him. When my son came home it was equally heart wrenching and I could not hide the truth from him. Jordan knew something was wrong and so we gently explained things to him, trying to reassure him that I would get better. However, inside I felt it was impossible and I had no positivity at this point, just the feelings of hopelessness".

These were extremely scary times and particularly traumatic for Sue, as we contemplated making our first steps implementing alternative approaches to fighting the cancer.

After being given little hope by the doctor, my wife and I sat down and discussed at length the details of the research I had been doing into alternative nutritional cancer therapies. I remember wrapping my arms around Sue in the kitchen and telling her everything was going to be ok, even though I felt inside like I had lost sight of the shore and swimming out in to unknown depths. However, in this moment I felt a distinct positivity that had been absent for what seemed like an eternity.

We both made the decision to take charge of the situation throwing everything into what I had researched and believed to make perfect sense. Nutritional therapy was a positive thing to do, having been told things were hopeless from a conventional treatment standpoint. This definitely gave Sue more hope and a positive focus which is in itself forms part of the healing process.

It really makes me cross when I hear people saying "you cannot give false hope to people", hope is hope and it is a good positive thing. Is it better when doctors pronounce what is in essence a death sentence of "you have three months to live"? These words are like voodoo and the doctors could be considered guilty of cursing someone to death by placebo. The power of the spoken word from such authoritative people in their white coats can be mighty indeed. Ask yourself which spoken words are more encouraging and beneficial to motivating people to better health and healing? I believe that hope is hope, hope is positive and positivity is influential in destressing and healing.

I will always remember speaking to one particular gentleman with cancer who was a friend of some friends of ours. We were invited to speak with him to explain what Sue had done having been written off by the medical establishment and that she no longer has cancer. We explained the importance of taking responsibility along with some of the strategies that we implemented. However he kept telling us; "you do not understand my cancer is different, my doctors have told me that I have three months to live". Nothing at all that we said would change his mind set as to the death sentence that had been cast over him. He had been through all the debilitating standard of care treatments and he had lost all his fight and all his hope.

Who knows he may have just simply been through enough which made him give in. We hear many stories of people going through the medical system which fails them and then as a last resort turn to natural ways to find that they get better, which is often referred to as 'spontaneous remission'. Who knows whether things could have been different for this man, had he taken control by implementing positive strategies into his diet, lifestyle along with detoxification etc. Basically to prevent feeding the cancer what it needed to thrive. Unfortunately this lovely guy passed away almost to the day of what the doctors had set for him. My experience and reality was that my mother, father, father in law, uncle and friends who had all gone down the cancer standard of care medical route had died.

> "Whenever a doctor cannot do good, he must be kept from doing harm."
>
> Hippocrates, Father of Modern Medicine

The first oncologist we saw at the hospital recommended performing biopsies of the stomach, liver and pancreas which we expressed our reluctance to allow. Through research, my understanding was that there were significant risks of metastasis (cancer spreading) when a tumour is punctured during a biopsy or cut into through surgery. The oncologist became rather unsettled at our reluctance to comply, but he did finally concede that there were risks of metastasis, but that it was a negligible two percent risk which in his opinion was quite acceptable. I simply could not rationalise this two percent figure with the knowledge that I had gained about the nature of cancer, as it just did not sit right in my mind.

When you consider the reality of what is being said here, this means that two people (real people) out of every hundred cancer patients (if these low quoted statistics are to be believed) will have their cancer spread further around the body through a biopsy. If you equate these figures to the 350,000 people who are diagnosed with cancer within the UK each year, then this means that potentially up to 6500 people may have their cancer metastasise through having a biopsy which is by no means an insignificant number.

My understanding was that the body builds a natural protein defence membrane around the cancer and if this is breached through surgical cutting, biopsy procedures or even 'high compression' breast cancer mammogram screening, then cancer cells are able to leach out and spread (metastasise) through the blood stream or the lymphatic system to seed in other locations throughout the body. The oncologist's manner became more authoritative and a little irate with our questioning and our decision not to authorise the biopsies of the tumours.

Further information from an oncologist confirmed privately to me that tumours in this location of the liver were usually of the most aggressive type, and statistically the prognosis was unlikely survivability. This deterioration would often happen quite quickly too, due to the tumour compressing and strangulating the vital bile duct tubes of the liver which in turn would prevent the liver from

No toxic chemotherapy,

No burning radiation therapy,

No surgery!

functioning properly to detoxify the body creating toxic build up and subsequent poisoning.

Subsequent scans and visits to the hospital which commenced six weeks into our strict nutritional therapy confirmed that the once

60 x 50 x 54mm tumour as seen on the original scan was now gone, leaving only 'scar tissue'. The three smaller growths on the pancreas were still there but the second oncologist we saw suggested that if we insisted in not to proceeding with biopsies at this time, then we would just monitor the situation and to come back if we found any further cause for concern.

We were sort of dumbstruck and the news did not seem to sink in straight away as to what we had just been told and what we had actually done. Of course there was still the uncertainty about the three tumours on the pancreas so we were still left with concerns, but this was without doubt fantastic news.

We are now over six years down the line and there have been no further stabbing pains or problems in the affected areas. Sue has put back on weight and we totally believe the significant changes we made in order to wreck the environment that was supporting cancer to thrive has proven its efficacy.

> "A control for cancer is known, and it comes from nature, but it is not widely available to the public because it cannot be patented, and therefore is not commercially attractive to the pharmaceutical industry."
>
> G. Edward Griffin
>
> Author & film producer of 'A World without Cancer'

To labour the point, because I cannot get enough of saying it, Sue's tumour is now totally gone and as the final oncologist we saw told us "only scar tissue of the tumour is left remaining".

The fact that scar tissue is remaining tells us also that it was not misdiagnosed, it was not a mix up in scans, the scar tissue left remaining is from a very real, sizable and dangerous tumour.

Dietary and lifestyle changes

What my wife Sue did was to follow a strict dietary change, which included plenty of 'raw organic' local vegetables, salads, herbs (live food) and spices which are well documented as anti-cancer fighting nutrition. The medical profession totally ignore what we now know to be crucial health information in nutrition and its tremendously influential role in cancer.

No conventional cancer treatment adds anything healthy or beneficial to building the body's already depleted immune system. What they do is to serve to further deplete the immune system through toxicity, burning and body tissue corruption in the hope that the cancer dies before the person. People are actually known to die of the

> **Pubmed study: Cancer is a Preventable Disease that Requires Major Lifestyle Changes**
>
> Published online 2008 Jul 15. PMCID: PMC2515569

common cold through the severity of the immune damaging effects of chemotherapeutic treatments.

To believe that cancer just happens in a genetic roulette without a cause as we are led to believe by the medical profession is to be at odds with the facts. It is like seeing the naked emperor and saying what spectacular and wonderful clothes he has, just because that is what everyone else is saying and we do not want to be going against the grain do we? I would encourage people to deeply question what is being said by the medical professionals and to think logically outside the box. I would also suggest to record meetings with healthcare professionals in order to take stock and revisit what has been said, as understandably it is difficult to take in all what is being conveyed in medical jargon language.

There were so many contradictions and questionable issues particularly with regard to my father's brain tumour and treatment that were later either denied or played down when we raised concerns.

My wife and I decided to take responsibility for ourselves, to do our own research and implement what we understood and believed to be sound common sense (albeit non-conforming) and who knows perhaps you may have to do this too.

The alternative is to surrender to everything that the doctors say, as gospel truth. This involves being treated with thirty year old chemotherapy treatments and one hundred year old radiotherapy (ionising radiation) which surely cannot be classed as cutting edge technology? The third part of the medical armoury is surgical butchery as a sledgehammer to treat cancer, which of course can be warranted in some immediate life threatening situations depending on the location of the cancer. All this whilst totally ignoring root causation which is significantly founded in poor nutrition, nutritional toxins, lifestyle and environmental toxins according to the World Health Organisation (WHO).

The first and foremost protocol we used was to cleanse the colon for a duration of ten days. The second protocol was to do a liver cleanse for ten days. It was important to do these processes in the correct order, firstly to create a clear pathway of elimination through the cleansing of the colon and then secondly to create an efficient liver through liver detoxification and supplementation of milk thistle. These simple procedures are discussed later.

We sourced good quality but simple dietary supplements.

We excluded all processed foods that man has synthesised or manipulated in some form or another, i.e. cakes, pies, pasties, burgers, sausages, reformed or reconstituted meat products, food colorants, preservatives, genetically modified foods, and sugars/sweeteners of all kinds.

We excluded red meat intake, fast foods or foods of convenience, along with taking out margarine, hydrogenated transfats and standard vegetable cooking oils which are well known to release cancer causing toxins when heated, especially repeatedly reheating oils at high temperatures. We took care not to cause browning or charring of any food which creates cancer causing acrylamides, so barbecued foods were definitely out.

Our rule of thumb was this, if man has been involved in processing the food product, or grown in corporate agriculture then we didn't touch it with a bargepole. We sought more natural or organically grown options, if it was not, we excluded it from our diet.

Our food choices may not always be perfect, but we can make better choices!

We eliminated dairy products from our diet which have been unhealthily processed by massive dairy corporations for extended shelf life and mass profit, not necessarily with our health in mind as people might like to think. The subject of milk is discussed later whereby you can reach your own conclusions.

We sourced and ate fresh vegetables which we consumed raw, steamed, or as lightly cooked as possible, because cooking destroys certain important nutrients and very importantly the natural enzymes which they contain. These natural enzymes are essential in supporting our digestive system thereby taking the strain off the pancreas and our body's inner resources.

Juicing is a fantastic way of ingesting raw fruit and vegetables and getting every last bit of goodness from them in an easily and fully absorbable form. Fruits and vegetables serve to alkalise the body's system, so are vital to us in creating healthy balanced and natural body chemistry.

Our strategy with Sue's cancer was to wreck the inner bodily environment that cancer needs to flourish through going back to basics. These basics included healthy natural alkalising and oxygenating nutrition full of vital minerals and nutrients essential for health.

We restricted higher sugar content fruit and starchy simple carbs (i.e. starch = sugar, sugar = cancer food) and this included the removal of processed and artificial sugars/sweeteners of all kinds.

Fruits such as apples, pears, or freshly squeezed lemons were the exceptions to this rule as they are low glycaemic (low in sugar). As a regular regime we juiced two green apples with a whole organic lemon (skin and all) and diluted in warm (not hot) water. This was fresh beautiful natural lemonade first thing in the morning with a hint of sweetness from the apples.

We also included pineapple and its stem due to its proteolytic enzyme (Bromelain) content which we understood assists in helping to break down proteins. We also understood Pineapple to have cancer fighting properties in the protease enzyme ability to digest protein of which cancer had a protein fibrin protective membrane. The degradation of the fibrin allowed the immune system cells to recognise and attack the cancer (ref: embryologist Dr John Baird). This was used in conjunction broad spectrum digestive enzymes and natural alkalising foods to assist in the cancer fighting armoury and changing the body's internal pH chemistry from acidic to alkaline.

Processed foods, over cooking, microwaves and the use of plastic cookware and film can denature food and create plasticization which the body struggles to recognise. The body then treats the food as a toxin and gives an alarm to your immune system which generates white blood cell activity to attack the denatured nutrients in a process called 'Digestive Leuko-cytosis'. This continual rallying to arms of the immune system serve's to set up the ground for auto immune diseases whilst depleting the body's energy and weakening the immune system.

This is not to say do not cook, but more to suggest care and the importance of including a fifty percent (plus) raw organic vegetation, salad or juicing into the dietary regime of a person who has cancer, just as we introduced into Sue's protocol.

We endeavoured to eat a wide variety of local organic or responsibly farmed vegetables. Sourcing organic produce would be fantastic if you are able to afford it, but if not, consider growing your own or sourcing produce from your neighbour's allotment or allotment society that you trust the way they grow food. Look for vegetables that are not grown with artificial/synthetic fertilisers,

> **Think of it this way**
>
> If the bacteria and bugs don't want to eat it then why would you?

or have pesticides, herbicide, larvicides, fungicides, or any growth stimulating chemicals sprayed on them.

Veggie boxes can be purchased from organic farmers or allotment societies in the UK Midlands area such as;

- **Riverford Organics,** Nationwide, UK.   Tel: 01803 762059
- **Trinity Farm, Cossall,** Nottingham, UK.   Tel: 0115 944 2545

These veggie boxes are naturally grown, local, seasonal produce just as we were meant to eat and they are great value for money. They can also be delivered right to your door.

Blending a variety of vegetables and then warming them up into a soup or perhaps a Stew, with natural raw Celtic sea salt or pink Himalayan rock salt, black pepper, herbs and spices is a wonderful way of getting maximum goodness into your system and not compromising on flavour. In general alkaline forming foods include: green leafy vegetables, cruciferous vegetables, most fruits, peas, lentils, beans, spices, herbs, seeds and almonds. Generally speaking acid forming foods include all meat, beef, lamb, pig, fish, poultry, milk and dairy, eggs, grains other Legumes excluding lentils and sugar. Acid forming drinks include fizzy soda pop, energy drinks, coffee, black tea, beers and spirits, pasteurized shop bought carton Juice.

The following is an excellent, but not exhaustive list of alkali forming vegetables that we included specifically in our cancer fighting and cancer preventative diet:

Natural Alkalising Produce

Chillie Peppers	Spinach	Leeks
Papaya	Broccoli	Shallots
Olives	lettuce	Chives
Chard	Cabbage	Peas
Dandelion greens	Runner beans	Sorrell
Tomatoes	Broad beans	Cucumber
Yams	Celery	Asparagus
Sprouts	Red Peppers	Kidney beans
Garlic	Cauliflower	Avocado
Ginger	Brussels	Lemons
Onions	Kale	Limes
Sauerkraut	Turmeric	Coconut
Carrots	Beetroot	Pineapple

Plenty to make beautiful stews, soups, and curry's etc. and the list is definitely not exhaustive.

We also included organic; brown whole grain rice, lentils, chick peas, quinoa, Almonds and other nuts and seeds. We removed white rice and white flour and white bread due to over refining processes and their starch content turning to sugar in the body.

We reduced the intake of simple carbohydrates with high starch pasta which turns immediately to sugar in the body. We 'reduced' high starch root vegetables like potatoes and took out parsnips due to high sugar as advised by our nutritionist.

These root vegetables are usually great for a normal healthy diet, but maybe unhelpful by contributing to the starch/sugar load when fighting cancer.

We included in moderation beetroot, sweet potato and carrots which have some wonderful nutrients for the body to utilise. Moderation and a balanced approach is the key here to creating your diet, and of course it is your decision. Carrots contain vitamin A and Beta Carotene which are known to have cancer fighting properties and fantastic nutritional benefits especially when juiced or eaten raw. Beetroot is also extremely good for cleansing the blood and fantastic juiced with green leafy vegetables and ginger.

We were of the opinion that many fruits being of higher sugar content especially over ripe may not be the best choice of foods to have whilst Sue had cancer. Organic apples and pears however which are low glycaemic (low sugar) fruits including their ground up seeds which contain vitamin B17 were acceptable choices. We also included lemons and limes which were low sugar and alkalising. The only other fruits we included were pineapple for the proteolytic enzyme bromelain content within the stem and some berries. If you do not have cancer then other preferably organic fruits are wonderful sources of nutrition.

Many Supermarket fruit and vegetables have been subjected to modern agricultural chemicals and mass industrial farming techniques which we understood to have toxic effects which gradually build up within the body through continued consumption. Often fruits, vegetables and salads are treated with radiation (irradiation) which prevents bacteria breaking down the produce and thereby giving more shelf life to the product. It is worth bearing in mind that in general the thinner the skin of the produce the more likely it is to be sprayed with pesticides and toxic chemicals.

The Dirty Dozen of chemical contamination

When it comes to taking out harmful toxins from your diet the following list might be very helpful. The 'Environmental Working Group' comprises of researchers, scientists, and policymakers who have developed a list of common produce items that have the highest amounts of pesticides and other harmful chemicals through 'non organic' corporate agriculture.

The Twelve Most Contaminated

- Apples
- Celery
- Cucumber
- Cherries
- Grapes
- Lettuce
- Nectarines
- Pears
- Peaches
- Potatoes
- Spinach
- Strawberries

> When purchasing any of the dirty dozen items then you might do well to get them organically sourced.
>
> Most of these you will notice are the thinner skinned produce which are usually more prone to chemical treatment and toxicity.

The Sugar/Cancer Issue

There is a large body of evidence in both medical and naturopathic fields that implicates sugar/glucose playing a significant role in the cause and subsequent feeding of cancer cells. Through our studies and reasoning we were in no doubt that we had to eliminate sugar and sugar inducing starchy simple carbohydrate foods from Sue's diet, which is what we did.

Sugar serves to acidify the body and greatly contributes to acidosis (over acidity of the body). As the second side of the same coin, the acidifying nature of sugar and most processed foods causes a depletion of the cellular oxygen, creating what is termed as an 'anaerobic' body environment (lack of oxygen). I understand that when sugar is introduced within these acidic, oxygen deprived cellular conditions that it promotes fermentation of the sugar which in turn changes the body's cells from the normal oxygen respiration to fermentation respiration (without oxygen).

These conditions shut down the body's normal cell functions which are intended to utilise life sustaining nutrients, oxygen and provide energy to the body. During the cells natural attempts to survive in these deoxygenated body conditions they go into out of control cell division and replication, cancer! The replicating cells become sort of immortal by losing their ability to switch off and die through their natural programmed cell death (apoptosis) and they continue to proliferate by dividing and splitting out of control.

There may be other issues that can be 'triggers' for cancer, but acidosis and an anaerobic bodily environment are essential underlying criteria for cancer and many other chronic diseases to develop. Triggers and contributors can be things like smoking, viruses, a bruise or cut, candida, auto-immune responses (i.e. the body attacking its self) or anything that kick-starts the healing process and immune system into gear.

Smoking serves to deplete cellular oxygen by blocking the lungs capacity to absorb oxygen and also causes the immune system to attack the toxins from the smoke and weaken or drain the immune system through continuously repairing biological damage.

This immune response to the cells being damaged may not switch off, causing cell proliferation and tumour growth. To understand this better think of the old saying 'the straw that broke the camel's back'. You could view this as the straw being the cause of the camel's back breaking, or if you sit back and think logically, the camel was already overburdened to the point of breaking and all it took was the straw which was the trigger. With cancer your body is overloaded and is in a prime disposition for cancer to develop and all it takes is to have the final straw to set it in motion, i.e. smoking, a bruise, candida, bacterial infection or emotional or psychological trauma etc. etc.

In 1931 Dr Otto Warburg won the highly prestigious 'Nobel Prize' for his pioneering works on cell respiration and cancer. Dr Warburg concluded that 'the prime cause of cancer is the replacement of the respiration of oxygen in normal body cells by the de-oxygenation, acidosis and subsequent fermentation of sugar within the bodily cells'. To my knowledge these scientifically acknowledged findings and conclusions have never been rescinded, but do appear to have been lost or ignored.

Just imagine this work was done all those years ago and yet this knowledge has not been utilised, even though Dr Warburg received the Nobel Prize for it. Some cynics might even say this has been suppressed by those who may lose financially were it to ever become common knowledge. The following is a seriously damning quotation from the Nobel Prize winning Dr Otto Warburg towards the cancer industry; it was taken from a lecture delivered to Nobel Laureates on June 30, 1966 at Lindau, Lake Constance, Germany.

"Nobody today can say that one does not know what the prime cause of cancer is. On the contrary, there is no disease whose prime cause is better known, so that today ignorance is no longer an excuse for avoiding measures for prevention. That the prevention of cancer will come there is no doubt. But how long prevention will be avoided depends on how long the prophets of agnosticism will succeed in inhibiting the application of scientific knowledge in the cancer field. In the meantime, millions of men and women must die of cancer unnecessarily".

As incredibly interesting and eye opening as this is, you do not need to understand all of the biological complexities of cells to know that this knowledge can be seriously considered in the armoury to fight cancer.

"The sugar industry has learnt the tricks of the tobacco industry. Confuse the public, produce experts who disagree, try to dilute the message."

Obesity expert Philip James

Our decision was to get rid of sugar' from many sources!!! However, the avoidance of sugar was not seen to be a silver bullet on its own, but this is what we considered to be a very important part of the overall armoury. We took out of our diet what we understood was in essence, one of cancers vital food sources, sugar, especially processed!

Artificial Sugars: There is a great deal of controversy over the safety of artificial sweeteners and there are many studies and evidences that say artificial sweeteners (Aspartame) have neurological health implications associated with them. Artificial sweeteners are also referred to as exito-toxins which are believed to stimulate brain cells to create a short term 'euphoria high' and enhancement of flavour, but in doing so they serve to progressively kill brain cells each time they are consumed. I believe that this is a gradual decline which goes unnoticed until symptoms start to appear whereby it may be too late.

I read from many sources that aspartame's neurological side effects are implicated in the following symptoms;

- Blurred vision,

- Headaches/migraines,

- Seizures/epilepsy

- Memory loss.

- Muscle cramps,

- Unsatisfied hunger (causing subsequent weight gain),

- Demise of kidney function

- Cancer.

Try Googling research carried out by the Neurosurgeon Dr Russell Blaylock and his findings and compare his research with any symptoms that you may have. I encourage anyone to research the dangers of Aspartame and draw your own conclusions.

With increasing awareness and concerns about the dangers of artificial sweeteners, aspartame artificial sweetener has now undergone a re-branding and is now being promoted as 'natural' would you believe.

The re-branded version of Aspartame is now called 'Aminosweet'.

Diet drinks and slimming foods often contain artificial sweeteners which are claimed to be healthier options due to zero calories for people trying to lose weight. Well the following information blows this myth right out of the water.

When artificial sweeteners are consumed the body makes preparations to receive that sugar rush that it believes is coming its way. The body releases insulin, the hormone which assists in the metabolisation and regulation of sugar in the bloodstream. Insulin helps to get the sugar out of the blood and into the cells for energy or to store it in fat.

However, although the sweetness from the sweetener has signalled for the release of insulin from the pancreas into the bloodstream, as there is no sugar/calories in the sweetener, insulin is released into the blood stream on a false alarm basis where it is not required. The insulin will do exactly what it is supposed to do and it will remove much, if not all of the remaining sugar from the blood stream and create fat cells in which to store it. The removal of these remaining sugars from the blood leaves the person hypoglycaemic, (low blood sugar) lacking in energy and craving for the replenishment of sugar and carbohydrates.

The person will then eat like there is no tomorrow as these food cravings are so powerful leading to over eating, weight gain and fat storage. The cycle is repeated each time these diet products are consumed which pile on the weight and pull the energy right out of the body. Can you see the logic of this?

If ever there was a case for breaching advertising standards, this would be it. Please check this information out and if you draw the same conclusions then I would encourage you to share this health enhancing information with your friends and loved ones.

Our decision to exclude aspartame/aminosweet and all similar artificial sweeteners was based on it being an unnatural synthetic product and our principle of ruling out processed foods and sugars of all kinds in our endeavour to change the bodily environment in which cancer thrived.

For your reference, aspartame is in almost every dilute juice and diet fizzy drinks in the supermarkets today. It is in chewing gum, processed foods, medications and also energy drinks with the double whammy effect of high dose caffeine.

Supplements, herbs and spices

Sue included the following supplements, herbs and spices

- Digestive Enzyme supplements,

- Acidophilus (Beneficial gut bacteria/flora)

- Sodium Ascorbate (vitamin C)

- Vitamin D3 with K2 (also obtained primarily from sunlight on the skin)

- Raw organic or home grown vegetables' and Salads,

- Freshly grown herbs, Parsley, Thyme, Rosemary, Mint, Coriander, Lemon Verbena, Nettles.

- Garlic, Cayenne Pepper, Turmeric/curcumin (in unison with Black Pepper), Cinnamon & Ginger Spices.

We invested in a weekly organic veggie box which is delivered to our door, as well as including nuts, seeds and berries, apricot kernels, small amounts of fish and chicken (white meat). We cut out red meat altogether, but now we have smaller portions of lamb and have it less frequently and we have cut out beef in general and all pork.

We detoxified the body and liver and cleansed the colon. These terms and products were all very unfamiliar to us at first and I understand that perhaps they may sound confusing to anyone who is unfamiliar, but it really was not too difficult. We also consulted a professional nutritionist who confirmed that we were very much on the right track. I would recommend anyone to work alongside a professional independent nutritionist or naturopath for guidance. The right professional will help you to work out your diet and help you to understand which supplements are important for you to have and why. Care should be taken when choosing a nutritionist as many of the medically sponsored nutritionists and doctors may not go much deeper than the limited concept of eating your five a day.

The more research I did, the clearer the picture seemed to become. This information was not selectively just for cancer, but serves to fuel and boost the body's own natural God given immune/defence system for all round health and wellbeing.

It is also about understanding the nutritional deficiencies and toxicity imparted into what we believe to be fresh healthy produce grown from modern corporate agricultural farming systems, which is discussed later in the book. In going back to basics and consuming local organic or responsibly farmed, live produce (vegetables, herbs, nuts, seeds, berries, legumes, pulses, fruits and salads) is to eat as nature intended and to guard against many westernised diseases like diabetes, heart disease, fibromyalgia, arthritis etc. and cancer.

"If prescription drugs are so great, then where are all the healthy takers"?

A visit to my doctor confirmed that I had arthritis in my hands and I was told that nothing could be done about this. I was told "well Robert you are of that age when this just happens". There was only talk of pharmaceutical drugs to manage pain and inflammation which all seemed to have disturbing side effects with long term use.

However my arthritis has now disappeared from my hands and the purple bone spurred knuckles are now normal. I accredit this to changing my diet to that of my wife's newly implemented anti-cancer diet which included raw organic vegetables, natural anti-inflammatory foods, detoxification and getting off the acidifying, deoxygenating, sugar laden artificial junk food. To term it another way, 'dead food'! I am amazed that the pain has gone from my fingers and I have found that I am able to play my guitar without discomfort.

In following and encouraging Sue's newly chosen lifestyle and eating regimen, I also lost two stone in weight, going from 15 stone 4 lb, to 13 stone 4lb, without any intention of losing weight in mind. Sue had become incredibly thin though, but it was interesting to see that she gradually started to put the weight back on that she had lost throughout her ordeal through the changes that we made. Additionally, I had suffered from rosacea for many years and had taken antibiotics and steroidal medication creams which had not resolved the problem. People would ask me if I had caught the sun which I became rather embarrassed about. After several years of this inflammation on my forehead, nose, cheeks and chest it has now gone too. I do believe the stress I had been under for a long time had a great deal to do with this issue as well, so de-stressing was also part of the regime of healing as well as optimum nutrition and removing toxicity.

> Cutting the cancer out, burning it out, poisoning it out in the hope that the cancer dies before the patient, seems to be the continuing medical approach to cancer!

The world famous quote of Hippocrates states; "Let thy food be thy medicine and let thy medicine be thy food". The medical institutes revered Hippocrates so much that they take the Hippocratic Oath to "first do no harm". I am in awe of the wonderful works that our hard working and passionate doctors do. I agree also that doctors are amazingly skilled in the field of medication and they are able to do fantastic works in A&E trauma etc. and lifesaving medicine. However, within disease control and long term treatments it appears that the medical establishment ignores Hippocrates most renowned quote of "Let thy food be thy medicine and thy medicine be thy food"!

Doctors receive very little training in nutrition, if any at all. This may consist of a mornings training to tip the nod on eating healthily, without really appreciating the full importance of nutrition over and beyond pharmaceutical drugs.

Many of our western illnesses can be attributed to nutritional deficiencies (orthomolecular) or toxic overload through our food. If I were to offer a pharmaceutical drug to address the symptoms of a starving man, what would you think? I hope that most rational people would see the logic of giving the man good constituted food as soon as possible. We have the paradigm of over fed people who are starving to death on a cellular level with our modern, addictive, flavour enhanced, artificial dead foods. Our medical institutes and government health agencies seem to have limited or low profile campaigns in the importance of education in preventative protocols for disease which addresses lifestyle and nutrition.

We have also seen some damning reports on various television programmes recently concerning the poor quality of food served to sick people in hospitals and even within our schools. Some hospital food that I witnessed left much to be desired in terms of its ability to nourish and build people up when they needed it the most during illnesses and convalescence.

A recent hospital experience of a very poorly member of my family was that the blood sugar levels were way too high and out of control. My step mother desperately wanted to get out of hospital, but was told that her blood sugar needed to stabilise before it would be safe for her to leave. I agreed with this wholeheartedly, but I had to ask how they planned on achieving this when I had witnessed processed foods, ice cream and apple pie being served which were in my understanding not conducive to achieving this aim. There was an uncomfortable mumbling of "this is not my area and not my fault", but I think the logic of my questioning struck home.

Cancer Research Funds,
Where do all the billions go?

In orthodox cancer treatment, doctors and oncologists are simply not allowed to step outside the realms of surgery (Cut) chemotherapy (cellular poisoning), or radiotherapy (radiation burning), which has gone unchanged as the three main core treatments for the past seventy years.

Literally billions upon billions have been raised for cancer research worldwide and this continues year in year out by generous hearted and well intentioned people. Think of all the races for life, the coloured wrist bands, supermarket cancer sponsorships, bungee jumps, parachute jumps, cancer donation tins, street charity collectors, party nights, boat races, charity shops, TV and radio campaigns, newspaper and magazine promotion, and online campaigns, all raising money for the cure for cancer!!!

For the last couple of years we have had the amazingly popular money spinning drive of Movember and Decembeard etc. etc. An incredibly clever and successful scheme dreamt up whereby men grow facial hair during a designated month to raise more money for the financially gorged cancer charities. There is now a no makeup cancer charity fund raiser as the latest money generator. Now imagine every village, every town, every city, every shire or state, then include every country 'worldwide' for over fifty/sixty years all working, giving, and donating to find the illusive cure for cancer at the rainbows end.

I wonder how many more people have to suffer the degrading and debilitating consequences before we begin to wake up to realise that it is impossible to find a medical 'Holy Grail' drug cure for a predominantly lifestyle and metabolically induced disease.

The cancer industry seems to continue to concentrate its efforts on what I view as the misguided track of early detection with the maximum of precision. This is then followed by the use of highly toxic patented drugs and treatments that by their own manufacturers material safety data sheets (MSDS) state that they cause cancer in humans.

Let us reflect on the treatments we continue to persevere with sixty to seventy years on. Yes, those very same highly invasive immune system damaging, toxic, carcinogenic (cancer causing) treatments of Chemotherapy, Radiotherapy, and surgery. Don't believe me that they are cancer causing? Types into your search engine the name of the drug in question followed by MSDS and download the material safety data sheet. Just to clarify for you, here are some of the medical terminologies used within the MSDS;

- Carcinogenic   = Cancer causing

- Category one   = Known to cause cancer in humans

- Category two   = Thought to cause cancer in humans

- Mutagenic   = Known to cause damage to the DNA of cells and damaging to unborn babies and young developing children.

I feel that each person should sit back, take stock and consider carefully the viability of cancer treatments that according to their own manufacturer's material safety data sheets are specified to cause cancer, in humans.

Everyone should know by now that ionising radiation causes cancer. Yet we use high doses of ionising radiation in mammograms, x-rays, PET scans and CT scans, and also radiotherapy in cancer standard of care treatments. Do these treatments really address the underlying issues of what caused the cancer in the first place?

Dr Benjamin Rush, a signer of the Declaration of Independence in 1776, fore sore a grim scenario that has now taken shape before our very eyes 238 years on.

Dr Rush claimed:

"Unless we put medical freedom into the constitution, the time will come when medicine will organise its self into an undercover dictatorship. To restrict the art of healing to doctors and deny equal privileges to others will constitute the Bastille of medical science. All such laws are un-American and despotic."

I think that the term 'mutagenic' and the skull and cross bones speak clearly for themselves.

Can we really believe that true healing can come from treatments that burn with radiation, poison with chemotherapy, make hair, teeth and nails fall out, destroy gut flora, gut linings and inhibit the ability to absorb nutrients and to vomit violently and profusely? Not to mention neuropathy nerve damage and sensory organ damage, which are considered acceptable collateral damage within the standard of care system? These treatments all serve to destroy the immune system which surely should be being boosted to fire on all four cylinders in order for the body's innate natural defences to fight disease, infection and maybe cancer too.

This is what I find incredible. We have placed men on the moon and missions to Mars. We have gone from computers the size of three story houses, to tiny microcomputers the size of pin heads with incredible power and capacity. We have gone from bi-planes to unmanned military planes that can travel 13000 mph (London to Sidney in one hour). We are well into what is known as the information age and we can speak to people the other side of the world face to face, plus we can have a clear understanding of genetics and the genome in how all things are made.

With all this in mind I would like to ask the question as to why it is that we are still using seventy year old plus, horse and cart technology of highly invasive, incredibly toxic treatments that according to the manufacturing pharmaceutical companies own material safety data sheets (MSDS) cause cancer? Insist that your doctor /oncologist gives you a copy of the material safety data sheet for these treatments, and be fully aware of all the facts to make informed decisions of what is the right path for you.

In this day and age, are these really the best cutting edge treatments that we have available after investing billions upon billions into cancer research? Ask your oncologist how old the drugs are that they are proposing to use because many chemotherapy drugs are twenty, thirty even forty years since they were developed. If this is the case then I would personally question whether this technology is really the cutting edge of science?

Remember by the World Health Organisation (WHO) and the various cancer institutes' own admission up to seventy percent of cancers could be prevented by better lifestyle and nutritional practices. Do we see the same passion to educate people from an early age on these preventative lifestyle factors as we see the passion to get people on to earlier and earlier treatments with the millions being invested into the recruitment drive of 'early diagnosis'?

In 1971 President Nixon publicly declared war on cancer and pledged to put whatever financial resources it would take to find the cure. Since then we have gone from one person in twenty, to one in two who will get cancer within their lifetime according to the Cancer Research UK (CRUK). Heads you win, tails you lose!

I am just so confounded in my thinking when I read that so many cancers could be prevented through diet and lifestyle and yet we see food and nutrition being largely ignored over what appears to me a race to recruit patients into the treatment system. Even now this drive continues as a treat it before it is even cancer, better safe than sorry! The latest trend appears to be using cancer causing' drugs like hormone blocking Tamoxifen as a cancer preventative treatment (ref; the manufacturers own material safety data sheets). Chemotherapy is even being used as a treatment for rheumatoid arthritis, What!!!

The concept I believe in treating rheumatoid arthritis with cancer treatment drugs is to knock out the immune system to prevent the body's natural immune response in attacking bodily toxicity displaced into joints (auto immune).

Well, my logic would dictate that we need to address the toxicity and remove it rather than suppress the immune response in attacking this build-up of toxins in the body. The arthritis may also likely to be the result of chronic long term dehydration, over acidity, processed foods, toxic load and inhibited detoxification through common western lifestyles.

Baring all of this in mind, my wife and I have taken the informed choice that we will never, ever, ever oh and did I say EVER, donate to any corporate engendered cancer charity whilst they appear to ignore logic and basic well known nutritional information in favour of continued use of highly toxic, but lucrative chemotherapy radiotherapy and surgery.

My Wife and I want to shout our experience from the roof tops, especially when I have witnessed and continue to see so many friends and family that are succumbing to these predominantly westernised illnesses.

I have personally met and spoken with many people written off by the cancer industry that have taken personal action and responsibility, implementing change in their lifestyle and diets, etc. whom no longer have cancer. My wife is now added to this list of people, by the grace of God.

Helping your body with nutrition not only assists in your physical wellbeing but greatly in your psychological wellbeing too. Your gut is also known as your second brain and if you are under nourished and nutritionally deficient, you will be more prone to: Anxiety, low mood, grumpiness, poor concentration, memory problems and depression too.

Cancer inhibiting or promoting

It was important for us to understand some basic facts about cancer and nutritional therapy in order to give confidence in what we were about to undertake. For Sue having cancer, we concluded that it was vitally important to have a well-planned dietary program to address the metabolic deficiencies and toxicity issues of the body developing cancer in the first place. This should be less confusing when you have an understanding of the basic principles of what you are trying to achieve with your body's internal environment in the fight or prevention of cancer.

Our Aims were to include the following;

- Cleanse the colon/bowels
- Detoxify the liver
- Parasite cleanse (wormwood, cloves, black walnut hull)
- Eliminate sugar, milk and dairy
- Juicing
- Eliminate processed junk food
- Alkalise the body and oxygenate the body
- Apricot kernels (B17)
- Keep the body well hydrated
- Take the strain off the immune system and support it
- Exercise and De-stress
- Supplements D3, K2, C, probiotics, enzymes, iodine etc.
- Adequate sleep
- Eat fresh, raw, organic, uncontaminated local produce
- Good natural oils (flax, extra virgin olive, coconut, avocado)
- Eliminate health & beauty toxins
- Remove environmental stresses and toxins
- Get back to home prepared cooking and no microwave

Within today's food culture we look to quick convenience and flavour as being major factors in what we choose to eat. This type of food is what should be referred to as dead food or artificial food which generally has very little nutritional value of which the body is desperately crying out for. This convenience foods are often one of the following or a combination of the following; highly acidifying, deoxygenating, dehydrating, toxic processed salt, unhealthy processed oils, loaded with sugars or artificial sweeteners, Mono Sodium Glutamate (MSG), absence of natural live enzymes and not forgetting; many are by design, highly addictive.

Processed foods have often been developed to contain taste enhancing MSG or other 'excito-toxins' like or aspartame (neuro-toxic artificial sweeteners) which are highly addictive and creates cravings for more carbohydrates and sugars. In addition there are also food colorants and preservatives, pesticides and other chemical residues and genetically modified foods which all serve cumulatively to alter the body's natural healthy environment and increase the build-up of toxicity, acidity and lower oxygen levels within the body. Prime conditions for dis-ease!

The Human body is an amazing thing in that it can tolerate many years of this sort of abuse, but sooner or later there has to come a time that something will break. The stomach may well be full, but the body lacks the vital fuel of vitamins, minerals, live enzymes and beneficial bacteria, that are necessary for a fully functioning immune system and healthy body.

Even if we eat supermarket purchased vegetables, salads and fruits, most people are totally unaware of the highly deficient nutritional value of modern day mass agricultural farming and the chemical toxicity they contain.

Our health, Soiled

Let's take a brief look at the soil: modern agricultural methods apply a synthetic fertiliser to re-mineralise the soil and feed the crops. These minerals are nitrogen, potassium and phosphates (NPK). However there should be more than seventy minerals present within the soil in order to grow fully healthy and nutritionally wholesome crops.

Our agricultural soils are becoming deserts, deficient of vital minerals and nutrients as a direct consequence of modern day mono crop intensive farming techniques. We therefore find that our crops are weakened and are more prone to attack from pests, bacteria, viruses and diseases.

Our poor farmers, frustrated and facing ruin go running to the chemical/pharmaceutical companies saying our crops are failing what can we do? The pharmaceutical companies are more than happy to solve the farmer's problems by supplying pesticides, herbicides-glyphosate, larvicides, fungicides and growth stimulants, to speak nothing yet about genetic modification and their far reaching health implications including nature and bio diversity.

There are too many people counting calories, not enough people counting chemicals!

So, many of the fresh vegetables and salads sold on our supermarket shelves are not only nutritionally deficient but are chemically laced, toxic food. Many of the pre-packaged salads are washed in toxic Chlorine and the plastic packaging may be pumped full of nitrogen gas' to preserve them from shriveling up in the natural process of aging.

Irradiation is also another highly questionable method of preserving fresh food produce which is basically radiation treatment. The radiation treatment prevents bacteria or pests from wanting to eat the food, but its ok for you to eat apparently.

Ask yourself, are all of these treatments serving to keep us in good health or are they ultimately for reducing wastage and increasing profit margins of the mass food corporations and supermarkets?

> Even the humblest creature has to know how to react to the difference between food and toxin if it's to survive....
>
> David Darling
> English astronomer & science writer

If the nutrients are depleted in the soil then they are deficient in the crops, so however much we eat and our stomachs feel full, our bodies will be nutrient deficient on a cellular level.

Please read back that last sentence again to ensure that you fully appreciate this simple but profound concept.

Due to the global nature of our economy much of our fresh produce is shipped in from overseas from several thousand miles away. This means that our so called fresh produce can be weeks if not months old, which in turn takes its toll in substantially depleting their nutrients even if they look perfectly fresh.

This is not meant to be all gloom and doom as Sue and I feel that armed with this knowledge will enable people to make better informed healthier choices. I cannot stress enough the importance of including fresh organic or responsibly farmed produce. People can take a stand against self-destructive unhealthy industrialized farming corporations that continue to use known harmful chemicals, fertilizers and genetically engineered crops.

We the consumer are able to make a stand by carefully considering where we choose to spend our money! Sue and I have taken the decision wherever practical, to support smaller local food producers, butchers and grocers. We try not to support the corporate supermarket monopoly's that in our view are leading the way in the overall demise in the quality of our foods eaten in society today

Interesting notes on cancer

- Dr John Baird, the well renowned Scottish embryologist and cancer pioneer published his papers in 1904 recognising that cancer was the body's natural healing process of cell reproduction/repair out of control. Dr Baird's studies found that this healing process went on to become cancerous when it was unable switch off by the normal bodily process of enzyme switching off action. Dr Baird studied this process and concluded that it was similar to the process of the placenta embedding itself into the mother's womb by trophoblast cells (cancer cells). He recognised that once the pancreas of the unborn baby starts to manufacture its own enzymes, these enzymes are then released, switching off the trophoblast (cancer) cells that have embedded the placenta safely and securely into the mother's womb.

- A benign tumour is a cancerous tumour that develops by the body's immune system having a delayed action in releasing the switching off enzymes at the repair site. This inhibited or delayed release of enzymes to the cellular damaged site allows the damaged cells of cancer to continue to develop before destroying them with the immune system cells or by programmed cell death kicking in (apoptosis). Many people have a misinformed, blasé opinion that a benign cancer is not dangerous or was never cancer at all. The so called benign tumour may not have developed the angiogenesis blood supply yet and full attributes as the malignant cancer, but it is still the body's reaction to harmful stresses in the bodily environment, toxic overload and psychological stress factors. It is also widely recognised that benign cancers can and do turn into malignant cancers, so it is clear that this is the same track process of cancer development. I also feel that the term benign can be used to discredit the effects of successful nutritional therapy which can turn cancer around, by being told the untruth that the tumour was benign and never cancer in the first place along with of course spontaneous remission.

- Cancer thrives within an acidic bodily environment, but struggles to survive in the body's normal mildly alkaline environment with a blood pH 7.365. Our whole cancer fighting concept and strategy was to wreck the bodily environment that cancer needed to thrive. We set out to starve cancer of what it liked and to give it what it did not like, in abundance. This we did by consuming healthy, organic, live, nontoxic natural foods, spices and supplements. However these guidelines are not limited just to cancer, it is also good advice for the many common chronic western auto immune illnesses where the immune system starts to attack itself, i.e. arthritis, MS, eczema, psoriasis, cancer, etc. It is about giving the body the tools to do exactly what God created it to do, to be healthy!

- This natural healthy blood pH of 7.365 may be strained by over consumption of acid forming foods which drive the body into the lower pH realm. The body will always regulate the blood pH otherwise you die and it will do this at the expense of using calcium from the bones to buffer, neutralise and regulate the blood pH. So, eating processed foods, foods of convenience, fatty foods, preservatives, colorants, high sugar content foods, reformed foods and excessive intake of meat all acidify. Many common drinks cause high acidity within the body especially fizzy sodas, alcohol and believe it or not milk (Casein protein and lactose sugar) along with its insulin like growth Factor (IGF1) hormones which are well known to stimulate cancer growth. Many of these foods contain what is called free radicals which are extremely damaging to the body's cellular structures; similarly to like rust being the damaging result of metal oxidisation. We can fight these free radicals by using anti-oxidants found in natural live foods, i.e. fruits, raw vegetables, fresh garden herbs, salads and various natural herbal teas, even dandelion and nettle teas.

- Cancer does not survive well in oxygen enriched bodily environments, but thrives in oxygen depleted environments. In 1932 Dr. Otto Warburg won the Nobel Prize for showing that cancer thrives in oxygen depleted environments (anaerobic). In other words, one of the main influences for the promotion of cancer is lack of cellular oxygen, acidosis (high acidity) and fermentation of sugars within this deoxygenated acidic body. A simple analogy is like comparing a healthy oxygen rich river teaming with life, to an acidic stagnant oxygen depleted pond which is full of stinking rancid bacteria. Are you beginning to get the picture?

- Interesting Note; there are eighteen cultures around the world where cancer and other westernised diseases simply 'do not exist'. These areas are termed as the Blue Zones. These cultures such as the Hunzakut tribe of the Himalayas, Abkhazians from Russia, Titicaca Indians from Peru or Okinawans from Japan regularly eat unadulterated raw vegetation, containing high density vitamins, minerals, chlorophyll and live enzymes, along with pure well mineralised water and living in a natural healthy environment. These people are renowned for regularly living in excess of one hundred years of age 'in extremely good health'. These are facts, but it is important that you confirm these truths for your selves! If this is true (and I personally am satisfied that it is), then westernised societies would do well to look into what these cultures are doing right. We should not be constantly firefighting disease which is running rampant through our society.

- The current cancer statistics in the western world are that one person in two people will get cancer in their life time, yet we are consistently told in the media and by orthodox cancer organisations and charity's that we are winning the war on cancer. If this is winning the war, I just dread to think what losing the war on cancer would be like! These articles are usually followed with statements like; the cure is just around the corner, we are pioneering new treatments, in the future, maybe, might, were not far away, the cure is on the horizon, then heart wrenching emotional stories are

> **CANCER**
>
> "Some 35 years of intense effort focussed on improving treatment must be judged as a qualified failure"
>
> John C. Bailar, MD New England Journal of Medicine, 1986

given which may well be genuine and true, but then to the clincher, 'but we need more money'. I was very sceptical when I first read about this and reluctant to believe, but then I started to pay more attention to all the cancer media hype and I have now built up a library of these newspaper and media articles. I can confirm that every one of them has this same theme running through them that the cure is just around the corner, we just need more money. Not only this, but there appears to be a blatant attack in discrediting herbs, nutrition and any natural concept outside of chemotherapy, radiotherapy and surgery. Mind those herbs and supplements, they might be bad for you, but chemotherapy, and radiotherapy that indiscriminately kill all cells, wrecks your immune system so you can die of the common cold and oh yes causes cancer are ok. I hope that you too will start to look at the wording within these articles and make your own minds up. The cancer statistics in the early 1920s were in the region of one in twenty people would get cancer in their lifetime. In subsequent years following President Nixon's declaration of war on cancer, hundreds of billions have been injected into drug intensive cancer research and they still appear to be procrastinating about the cause. The worldwide cancer business is worth 500,000,000000 (half a trillion dollars a year). However the same highly invasive toxic cancer treatments remain predominantly unchanged with more and more people than ever succumbing to cancer who are being perpetually treated, treated and treated.   One person in two!!!

- There is much evidence for the therapeutic value of many naturally occurring nontoxic foods, herbs spices and supplements which actively seek out and destroy cancer cells or that create a body environment that is hostile to cancer. I read that Vitamin C has a powerful anti-cancer action by eating fresh organic fruit and vegetables, vitamin supplementation, or even through mega dose intravenous vitamin C. Linus Pauling two times winner of the Nobel Prize and one of the greatest biochemists of modern times fully endorsed the use of vitamin C as a valuable anti-cancer aid. Pauling became unpopular within the medical realm and was criticised and attacked due to his outspokenness about the cancer industry. No one can argue about the genius mind of Linus Pauling. Turmeric has the active component curcumin and there is an abundance of scientific studies affirming its highly anti-cancer properties, especially when taken in unison with 'black pepper'. The bio active availability increases a thousand fold when curcumin is taken with black pepper. Dark green nitrosilic foods like Spinach, Kale, dandelion leafs, wheatgrass, sprouts and shoots, along with cruciferous vegetables Broccoli, cabbage, Brussel sprouts, cauliflower etc. are also widely recognised for their highly anti-cancer properties, especially when juiced or eaten raw.

- Foods containing vitamin B17 are also renowned to have cancer fighting properties. Some of these foods include the following: apple seeds, pear seeds, apricot kernels, Peach nuts, blackberries, tapioca, grasses, shoots, millet. Sue ate approximately around 35 apricot kernels per day, 5 or 6 at a time, every couple of hours or so. Sue did not initially like these nuts and I noticed that she was sneakily swallowing them whole without chewing. I had to explain that she must chew them to a pulp in order to get the full benefits from them. The apricot kernels could be grated and sprinkled on oats or over other foods to disguise the bitter flavour. Some people soak the nuts overnight to make them easier to eat and more readily broken down. Dr Ernst Krebs pioneered research into Vitamin B17 and its other forms; Laetrile, Amygdaline to prevent and to fight cancer. It was important for us to ensure that we purchased the 'bitter apricot kernels', not the sweet variety which do not contain B17.

The armoury of going into battle

I hope that you are beginning to understand how we changed Sue's bodily environment to be hostile to cancer. Simply based on the information above, we knew we had a great guide as to how we were able to fight against cancer and give Sue the best chances of overcoming it. Let's run through these concepts.

Alkalising the body.

Firstly it was important to address the pH of our body's internal environment from too acidic where cancer thrives, to alkaline in which cancer does not thrive. This was done by eating what is known as alkali ash foods (foods that impart an alkalising residue within the body) i.e. fresh, local, organic or responsibly farmed vegetables and salads as near to their fresh and natural state as possible. Introducing raw salads and vegetation (live foods) also serves to keep the body well oxygenated because to be in an alkaline state means that the body is able to absorb more oxygen on a cellular level and we know that cancer prefers a de-oxygenated environment. Eating raw natural foods also assists in maintaining essential good gut flora (healthy stomach bacteria) along with the natural live enzymes from the raw vegetation. The skins of vegetables and fruits also have antibacterial, antifungal, antiviral phytonutrients which the body uses to on a cellular level. Many cancers can be caused through pathogens getting into cells and damaging mitochondria, DNA and switching off apoptosis.

It was a revelation to find out that when we cook vegetables we kill the live enzymes and significantly deplete many nutrients which are so important to our body's health and fighting against disease. This is not to say that we should not cook vegetables, but that we tried to include at least 50% and above raw organic vegetables and salad produce in to our cancer fighting dietary regime.

Water/hydration.

We purchased a basic activated charcoal water filter jug and drank plenty of fresh pure water 1.5 to 2 litres per day to help the body to process food and to flush out toxins efficiently. We chose not to drink water during mealtimes because this would serve to dilute stomach acid and enzymes which would inhibit digestion. Drinking cold water with meals also inhibits enzyme-biological actions which work optimally at warm body temperatures. Eating ice cream after a meal will also serve to inhibit digestive enzymes, allowing unbroken down indigested foods through into the small intestines and subsequent mal-absorbsion. You can also consider putting a teaspoon of bicarbonate of soda in a glass of water once or twice per day to help alkalise the body thirty minutes before or an hour after food.

<u>Building the immune system Empowering Digestion.</u>

We should look to re-introduce vital foods or supplementation of vitamins and minerals that are largely missing from our normal diet due to processed artificial foods, modern day intensive farming and soil depletion, not to mention further depletion through cooking our natural live foods to death.

Probiotics build and create good gut bacteria (gut flora) within the digestive system which assists the body's ability to digest, break down and assimilate food into the body. Probiotics create a healthy digestive system and build the overall immune system. The probiotic supplement that we chose was 'acidophilus'.

Why eating fermented food is good for health

The process of fermentation of food goes back thousands of years and the benefits to health can be nothing short of amazing.

Since the dawn of time fermenting foods has provided man with a highly effective way of preserving fruits, vegetables and meat as a means of storing up food for times of shortage.

The Fermentation process occurs under deoxygenated conditions; which allows anaerobic bacteria and enzymes to biologically break down food. This biological break down pre-digests food which serves to assist the body in digestion making it readily assimilated into the body.

The process also promotes healthy live bacteria which is vital and a fundamental part of our gastro intestinal wellbeing. This good bacterium (gut flora) contributes up to eighty percent of our immune system and fermenting foods is a natural way to generate this healthy gut flora of probiotics. This can be a major advantage in building up the immune system when dealing with chronic disease.

Fermented foods are particularly important whilst taking antibiotics as antibiotic medications indiscriminately kill all bacteria in the body, both beneficial and bad bacteria. It is therefore vitally important to reintroduce and encourage good gut bacteria into the body following these medications.

We can increase good gut bacteria by eating fermented vegetables of all kinds, such as sauerkraut, coconut kefir, Kimchi, and Kombucha. These products were taken in addition to using acidophilus probiotic supplementation.

Digestive Enzymes

We supplemented with digestive enzymes to assist the body in the efficient breakdown of food nutrients. Supplements should be sourced from reputable companies and made from natural substances **NOT** cheap artificial, synthetically produced with caking agents, artificial sweeteners and bulking fillers like many found in supermarkets today. Other ways of introducing digestive enzymes are to eat raw organic fresh vegetables, salads and to include green juicing.

Making better food choices.

Most importantly we reduced or took out of our diet, foods that are known or implicated in the promotion of cancer cell growth. We removed processed foods, reformed foods, red meat, pork, reconstituted/reformed meats, genetically modified foods and foods containing preservatives, colourings and flavourings and other additives. Additionally modified fats, margarines and processed sugar content products.

House of Commons Food Procurement Policy

"In line with its procurement policy, the House of Commons Catering Service avoids, wherever identifiable, the procurement of foods that contain genetically modified organisms,"

This is from a statement in the U.K. Parliament's own restaurant food procurement document.

"To this end, as part of the tendering process, food suppliers are required to work to a strict GM organisms policy and give assurances that goods supplied be free from genetically modified materials."

I find it interesting that we are told by our government that GM foods are perfectly safe and nutritious for us. However the recent 'procurement policy' for MPs within the House of Commons stipulates to its suppliers organic non GMO food procurement only!

Hmmm, what's good for the goose apparently is not in the House of Commons view good for the gander!!!

To cook or not to cook.

We should also understand that the longer we cook vegetables the greater this influences the depletion of their nutrients. Lightly steaming or shorter cooking times would help to retain more of the natural nutrients in cooked vegetables that our bodies desperately require for good health.

Look at it this way, whilst our bellies may be full and satisfied our body and especially our immune system could be seriously compromised and depleted of essential nutrients to keep you disease free and healthy. It simply makes perfect sense to source the best organic foods to enable our bodies to do what they are designed to do given the right conditions and nutrients, this being, to be healthy, fight disease and heal itself.

The skins of fruits and vegetables contain antibacterial, antifungal, antiviral and anti pest phytochemical/nutrients. When we eat these God given phytonutrients our body can utilise them for its own protection against harmful pathogenic invaders.

Over cooking actually causes plasticisation of the foods and the body generates white blood cell activity (digestive leukocytosis) whereby the immune system kicks into gear to attack the very food that is supposed to nourish it.

Ensure that you have plenty of raw unadulterated salads, vegetables, and juicing as well as cooked and natural oils. Remember that If you have cancer then the diet to consider would be at least fifty percent and above raw vegetation content. Just bear in mind that doctors are there to treat mainly symptoms us when we are broken, but it is our job to ensure we do not break in the first place.

Lemon-aids health

Lemons are a rich source of vitamin C, B vitamins, riboflavin, along with minerals like phosphorus, calcium, magnesium as well as antioxidants and dietary fibre. Lemons are low glycaemic (low sugar) and therefore low in calories, being one of the lowest among the citrus group. Lemon juice consists of about 5% citric acid which is a natural preservative that gives the tart taste to lemon.

The best time to take lemon water

Whilst you may drink lemon water any time of the day, drinking lemon water first thing when you wake up has wonderful health benefits. Your body is literally on a fast whilst you are asleep and is in a mildly dehydrated state when you awake in the morning. Lemon water re-hydrates your body within minutes, unlike coffee which is loaded with the diuretic caffeine; this takes more fluid from your body in order to process it. Lemon juice is a great way to energise quickly in the morning. It is less sugary than orange juice and a great healthy, refreshing and economic way to wake up to in the morning!

Why drink lemon water?

1. Boosts immune system: Because of its rich Vitamin-C content, lemon water strengthens your immune system and helps prevents colds and various illnesses and we used lemons in part of the armoury of our anti-cancer diet.

2. Supports the digestive system: Lemon water helps your liver to produce bile which digests fat for easier absorption of fat soluble vitamins.

3. Promotes clear skin: Your body's inner health is directly reflected through the condition of your skin. Depending on what you feed your body, what you eat or drink may nourish or be harmful. Drinking lemon water effectively cleans your bowels of harmful waste and toxins so that with regular consumption, your skin will look and feel healthy and blemish-free.

4. Lemons create the feeling of satiation and taking away that feeling of hunger which assists with weight loss.

5. A regular intake of lemon water promotes an efficient elimination process, and lemons assist in lowering the absorption of sugars from the food you eat.

6. There are more nutrients within the skin of the lemon than actually in the juice, so juice the whole lemon with your green juices to give them a zing.

6. Although the lemon is acidic when consumed the residual effect to the body (the ash) is highly alkalising perhaps one of the most alkalising beneficial fruits you can eat.

B-17 Apricot Kernels,
(AKA Vitamin B17, Laetrile or Amygdaline)

Alongside changing to a healthier more natural diet, foods containing vitamin B17 are renowned to have amazing properties in fighting and preventing cancer. Apricot kernels/pits are predominantly one of the most well-known source of vitamin B17, however apple, pear, peach, cherry pips/nuts, blackberries, blueberries, tapioca pudding and millet flour all have vitamin B17 or B12 cyanates in them (cyanide). Various studies have shown the use of vitamin B17 selectively attacks and kills cancer cells.

The science of how this works. Vitamin B17 contains two molecules of glucose, one molecule of benzaldehyde and one molecule of hydrogen cyanide (HCN). Many people recoil taking a sharp intake of breath when the word cyanide is mentioned and quite rightly so, in its free & synthesised form. However there is 'no free' hydrogen cyanide in Apricot Kernels (vitamin B17, or Amygdaline) as this has to be manufactured by a certain enzymatic process to release it within the body.

There is an enzyme called beta-glucosidase that is found present 'only' at the cancer site which has the unique ability to unlock and unleash the cyanide and benzaldehyde directly at the point of the cancer cells. Because there are two molecules of glucose within the B17 these are drawn straight to the cancer as cancer cells have at least ten times more glucose/sugar receptor sites. The 'PET/CAT scan' takes advantage of this fact which places radiated sugar into the body which acts like a Trojan horse into the cancer cells. The cancer cells then glow up like a light house on the scan. The B17 is broken down by the betaglucosidase enzyme to free the hydrogen cyanide and benzaldehyde molecules which poison the cancer cells, similar to the action of a targeted heat seeking missile and is perfectly nontoxic to normal cells.

The key thing to realise here is that the Hydrogen Cyanide 'must be formed' and is unable to form without the unlocking enzyme beta-glucosidase. This enzyme and only this enzyme, is capable of manufacturing the Hydrogen Cyanide from B17 within the body. If there are no cancer cells in the body, there is no beta-glucosidase, if there is no beta-glucosidase, no free cyanide will be formed from the vitamin B17. This is a natural target specific way that is found in nature which I find absolutely incredible. The enzyme Rhodanese is abundant throughout the body except at the point of cancer. Rhodanese is involved in cyanide detoxification and converts the cyanide into Thiocyanate and benzaldehyde into Benzoic acid which are beneficial in nourishing healthy cells and forms the production of vitamin B12 in the body.

Vitamin B17 does contain the cyanide radical (CN). This same cyanide radical is contained in vitamin B12, and in berries such as blackberries, blueberries and strawberries. You never hear of anyone getting cyanide poisoning from B12 or any of the above-mentioned berries, because they do not.

Sue ate thirty to thirty five apricot kernels per day, but not all in one go! Sue took about five or six at a time throughout the day and making sure they were well chewed. I understand that anyone who chooses to eat the kernels as a preventative measure would probably take about six to eight kernels per day. The kernels can be grated and sprinkled over other foods which enhance the beautiful almond flavour and disguise the bitter overtone. I must emphasise that we ensured that we had the 'bitter apricot kernels', not the sweet alternative that do not contain vitamin B17. We gradually just got used to the bitter flavour of these little nuts.

For a more detailed analysis of the theory and science behind B17/Laetrile and its use against cancer cells, see G. Edward Griffin, 'A World Without Cancer' (Thousand Oaks, CA: American Media,

1974). A video presentation can also be viewed on the internet via 'Youtube'. You can also research Dr Ernst Krebs Junior who pioneered research into vitamin B17. Another great book is: B17 Metabolic Therapy, by Phillip Day of Credence Publications.

Please be aware that there has been a mass smear campaign against these apricot kernels and the people who have been instrumental in their research. Bringing public attention to the science behind Vitamin B17, apricot kernels, Laetrile and Amygdalin is a precarious business.

Apricot kernels contains Benzaldehyde, a natural analgesic (pain killer) which I read has the effect of reducing the pain of many cancer sufferers when taking them. Many cultures the world over eat foods rich in vitamin B17. Earlier this century within the UK we had Millet as one of our staple grains which contained B17, but as our modern culture advanced, wheat was introduced and now Millet is virtually unheard of.

The Hunza tribe from the Himalaya's prize their apricot Kernels as a staple part of their diet and have done so for thousands of years. It is interesting to note that not one case of cyanide poisoning has been documented through eating these kernels that I am aware of. It is also worth noting that these cultures do not suffer the degenerative diseases such as cancer, sugar diabetes, heart disease etc. that our westernised societies do.

Some people on occasion say that they feel a little off when they have been taking the kernels and this might well be because the B17 is doing its job as it is supposed to do. When the cancer is under attack and the cancer cells start to progressively die, these cells have to go somewhere and they

Important: If you have a compromised liver function, then further professional guidance is advisable when undergoing any form of detoxification process including taking B17 in order to prevent overloading a poorly functioning liver.

have to be taken out of the body through the channels available to them. This can cause burden on the liver especially if the liver is compromised and is not functioning efficiently.

However there is striking a balance between feeling a little off and over burdening the liver. From feedback I have received, most people are perfectly ok as Sue was, but if in doubt ease back on the kernels and build them up gradually and or seek professional guidance.

Some people soak the kernels for a few hours to make them softer and easier to chew and digest.

I have tried to maintain a balanced approach by learning about all aspects of the story concerning vitamin B17 apricot kernels, Amygdalin and Laetrile. I have to say that I am really surprised that my wife and I are still alive based on the information on the 'Cancer Research UK' (CRUK) website which reads as follows:

Quotation from 'CRUK's' website 2013:

"Laetrile (amygdalin, vitamin B17) Side effects"

*"Laetrile contains cyanide, which is a type of poison. So the side effects of laetrile are the same as those of cyanide. These include" Sickness, Headaches, Dizziness, Liver damage, A lack of oxygen to the body tissues, A drop in blood pressure, Drooping eyelids, Fever, Nerve damage, causing loss of balance and difficulty walking, Confusion, coma and eventually **death"**!!!*

All I am able to say is that this has not been our experience when taking vitamin B17, having eaten thousands of apricot kernels alongside my wife during and following her skirmish with cancer. I have to wonder why CRUK uses such 'scaremongering tactics' which serve to put many people off using the apricot kernels.

I have had the pleasure of meeting and speaking with so many people with cancer, some whom had been written off by the cancer industry who are still alive today 'without Cancer' simply by modifying their diet and including apricot kernels (vitamin B17) in their new dietary regime. We have just received news of a lady who had a brain tumour the size of a plum who made the personal decision to eat the apricot kernels. This lady recently got in touch to let us know that she no longer has the tumour, having altered her diet and having included apricot kernels. I also believe totally in the power of prayer and know that many prayers were said for her.

I find CRUK's stance on B17 very interesting, but also bewildering based on our practical experience and what I would consider wholesome, innocent little nuts. Maybe I am nuts though!

Sue and I exercised care and common sense in the amounts taken of course, but the same would go for eating too many dry roasted peanuts, just be sensible.

Look at this analogy; Water is good and essential to us for life but try to drink too much to quickly and you will drown!!! Does this mean water is bad for us, no, it means be sensible!

I have a friend who has been eating apricot kernels for the last sixteen years and somehow she is still alive. How the Hunzakut tribe of the Himalayas ever survive to well in excess of 100 years of age eating these apricot kernels as a staple part of their diet, you will have to make your own minds up. Remember also that bitter foods have largely been removed or bred out from our diets because sugar and sweetness sells and there is more profit in sweeter things.

Meat

Ingestion of Meat

It takes massive quantities of pancreatic juices and digestive enzymes to liquefy and digest meat, particularly red meat. Additionally the energy that this digestive process takes from the body is considerable, especially when the body needs to conserve as much of its energy and resources as possible for fighting the cancer.

Meat also serves to acidify the body, so therefore we felt it to be vital for us to exclude especially red meats from the diet of a cancer sufferer. We also considered it to be important to reduce the intake of white meat (chicken and fish) to palm of the hand sized portions should you have cancer. It is worth noting that by depleting the massive amount of pancreatic enzymes required to break down meat renders your body deficient of enzymes which are also required for many other functions within the body and potentially in breaking down the protein fibrin coating surrounding cancer cells for the immune system to recognise the uncloaked cancer and send in the infantry.

Pork, is from a scavenger beast

Pork is a meat that is found in different forms and dishes, i.e. Bacon, Sausage, Ham, luncheon meat, black pudding and Gammon. A pig is a scavenger beast and can tolerate eating all kinds of putrid foods that normally could not be tolerated by most other animals. Pigs do not have sweat glands for expelling toxins and they are known to store these homo-toxins within their body and are also highly prone to microscopic parasitical life forms which can be directly transferred into humans during the consuming of pork.

These microscopic parasites trigger the body's immune system creating white blood cell activity against them and thereby depleting the body's defence resources in fighting against them. Additionally it is known that you have to be very careful with pork due to it going off very rapidly, especially in warmer climates. The parasite issue within pork can be passed into humans who ingest the meat and parasites are believed to be a contributory factor in triggering some cancers. Within wise scripture it warns people with good reason against eating swine as it is termed unclean.

Pork is also acidifying to the human body's environment, takes resources from the body so these were reason enough for us to remove pork from Sue's anti-cancer dietary regime.

Red meat

Red meat in particular takes a great deal of the processing resources of our digestive system. Red meat also takes a prolonged time to go through the digestive system and bowels and the longer it takes for food to go through our system the more prone it is to Putrefaction.

This Putrefaction builds up within the gut intestines/bowels whereby the resultant toxicity is re-absorbed back into the body through the intestinal wall, creating numerous potential health problems and a forerunner to disease.

Meat products are one of the main reasons why we get intestinal worms and parasites and these place an enormous strain on the body and the immune system. Many of the nutrients from our foods can be consumed by these parasites leaving your body further nutritionally depleted. Our immune system also has to deal with the toxic waste that parasites dump into our body.

I understand that the start of many degenerative diseases originate within the bowels. Our aim should therefore be to get the bowels moving regularly and efficiently to prevent putrefaction, bowel plaque build-up and generally clogging up the system at all cost.

Fish

Oily fish (Salmon Mackerel, Sardines, Herring Trout, Pilchards, Kipper, and Anchovies) are a good source of omega 3s and in moderation can be eaten by cancer sufferers. Fish can be an excellent source of Vitamin D which is highly anti cancerous and it is well established that most cancer sufferers are deficient in vitamin D.

Deep sea fish Cod, Haddock, are also an option in moderate quantities. Fresh water fish like trout are also excellent choices. Try to steer clear of mass farmed fisheries due to man messing around with the natural way of things with growth stimulants, antibiotics and GM foods fed to these fish. The fish should not be fried, battered, smoked or preserved in any way.

Chicken

Chicken is a white meat and is generally easier for the body to digest in comparison to red meats. The source of any meat consumed is of vital importance in terms of its healthy nutritional content or potentially harmful toxicity. Hens sold by large supermarket outlets and fast food corporations are generally sourced from intensive farming outlets.

To those who have a heart for the pain and misery of animals, this modern day farming is inhumane, unnatural, and unhealthy, what I would consider atrocious rearing conditions. Chicken factory farms have been slammed by the RSPCA with new research identifying cruelty on a massive scale. Tens of millions of weak and injured 'factory' birds die every year because their bodies cannot cope with regimes designed to speed their growth and the drugs and antibiotics routinely fed to keep them from disease in filthy unsanitary and cramped conditions. It almost reflects the evil and disgraceful black slave trade of packing them in like sardines, in what can only be described as a hell on earth.

> **RSPCA exposes horror of intensive chicken farming**
>
> Mail Online, Friday, Jan 17 2014

Birds sourced from these conditions are laced with routine antibiotics, growth hormones or stimulants for bulking up in half the time of natural growth. I suggest researching the factory farming of chickens and the disease and death rates that are the norm. We opted for organic or responsibly reared chicken wherever possible.

I think that it is only right that if we are to take the life of an animal for our consumption then we should treat it with dignity and respect in its keeping. Another way of looking at it would be that the animal from its death may have the last come back on you.

> If you eat unhealthy
> you become unhealthy
>
> **You are what you eat!**

If you are eating intensively farmed, toxin laden meats, stressed and sick animals then you may soon find somewhere down the line there are consequences and that people may become toxic, stressed and sick. We are what we eat is a commonly used phrase.

Milk & Dairy produce

We were fairly strict with cow's milk and dairy, taking out most dairy produce. No Cow's Milk, Cheese or yogurts laced in sugar, however we did have small amounts of 'organic' butter from grass fed cows.

We changed to healthier option milk such as; coconut milk, rice milk and homemade almond and cashew nut milk which were wonderful. It was just a case of getting used to something a little different when you know it is part of the armoury to regaining health. Do not see this as just taking all the things that you love away, see it as introducing wonderful replacements that are different but will serve you and your health better. You will be amazed how after twenty one days your palette and your old habits will change to your newly found nutrient enriched options.

We understood that Goats Milk although not ideal due to its natural hormones and processing, was more easily assimilated into the body than cow's milk and therefore maybe a better choice. However we chose not to have it for Sue as we took out animal milk all together.

Milk today is not the same milk as when I was a child. I remember milk going off by the following day of being delivered, which was perfectly normal as we had milk delivered fresh every day.

I remember having to beat the sparrows to the milk before they pecked into the silver foiled bottle tops to access the beautifully rich unadulterated cream floating on the surface. In contrast my wife and I recently observed a bottle of green top milk that lasted for over two weeks. I have to ask, is this same milk as my childhood days?

Milk goes through unnatural processes of sterilisation and homogenisation at super-heated temperatures and incredible pressures which kill off all enzymes and bacteria both good and bad. In fact it kills off anything biological that might have been beneficial to the body. These processes change the milk at a molecular level and make it difficult for our bodies to recognise this plasticized product that is no longer in its natural state.

Milk is also contaminated with growth hormones, 'Insulin Growth like Factor One' (IGF-1) lactating stimulants, routine antibiotics and steroids which come directly into our food chain by the consumption of dairy. These chemicals and drugs are all used in what I see as short term profiteering by massive corporations who do not seem to take into consideration the pain and suffering to the poor beasts and also the long term health effects to us as consumers who have many allergic reactions to milk. Is this really good daily nourishment for us and our children?

With the unnatural and unhealthy living/rearing environments the beasts often suffer from diseases and infections like mastitis, causing blood and somatic cells (puss) to be excreted and contaminated within the milk through this factory production line system. There is apparently a legally acceptable 3% level of somatic puss cells allowable in your milk that you drink day in day out. It sure puts you right off your milky porridge in the morning.

Insulin Growth Factor - 1 and Cancer.

"The IGF signalling pathway has a 'pathogenic role in cancer'. Studies have shown that increased levels of IGF 1 [*contained in milk and dairy products*] lead to increased growth of existing cancer cells"[21]

76

Hematol Oncology Clinic North America. 2012 Jun;26(3):527-42, vii-viii. doi: 10.1016/j.hoc.2012.01.004.

Epub 2012 Feb 28.Targeting the insulin growth factor receptor 1.

This was as clear as day to us, we needed to come straight off dairy products!!!

> ## Insulin like growth factor Raises Cancer Risk
>
> By William J. Cromie
> Harvard University Gazette, April 22 1999
>
> High levels of a well-known growth factor significantly increase the risks of colorectal, breast, and prostate cancer, medical researchers have found

It is an unbelievable revelation when your eyes are opened and realise just what is happening to our milk and how it affects the body. I also understand that milk manufacturers are now putting sugar and artificial sweeteners (Aspartame) in milk and dairy yogurts in their endeavours to tempt our taste buds and increase milk sales, especially to children.

There is a great deal of research to implicate aspartame as being a highly damaging neurotoxin, which excites and stimulates brain cells so your 'feeling' and 'taste' sensations are enhanced, but then the exitotoxin progressively kills off those brain cells. There is a very interesting documentary film called 'Sweet Misery' which you may find very interesting on YouTube or to purchase the DVD.

In brief, for cancer sufferer's, the high protein (casein) and milk sugar (lactose) content in milk and dairy products promote an acidic body environment 'acidosis'. The lactose is milk sugar and we know that cancer is a sugar metaboliser. Are we therefore not contributing directly to providing a bodily environment for cancer to thrive, ref; Otto Warburg's Nobel Prize for establishing this. Milk sugar (lactose, galactose) also directly serves to feed the cancer as the cancer is an optimum glucose metaboliser. In addition to this the growth hormone, 'Insulin Growth Factor One' contained in milk and its cancer promoting qualities were all reasons enough for us to take

> I read a study stating: If young babies are bottle fed with cow's milk, they may suffer from hardening of the arteries and high blood pressure later in life, leading to potential coronary heart disease.

dairy products out of our diet, especially as a cancer sufferer.

Milk production has turned into a 'production line' industry of mass profit. According to my research studies, cows are administered steroidal growth hormones in order to fatten up the calves quickly and to increase mother's milk production with lactation stimulants. These female oestrogen hormones come directly through the milk into our food chain from our early childhood as the authorities promote milk to our young children at school saying that it is good for bones and teeth.

These, often synthetic hormones are not too dissimilar to human oestrogen and it is quite frightening to think of the long term implications that these may have on humans alongside the xenoestrogen hormone disrupters in plastics. We are seeing young girls coming into puberty at an ever increasingly younger age (seven to nine years of age instead of twelve to thirteen). We are now seeing more and more gender altered/confused issues within males in our society as never witnessed to this extent before.

Xenoestrogen activity from unnaturally occurring man influenced processes like our overabundance of plastic are also known to influence cancer and also normal male sexual traits by over dominance of the female hormone mimicking oestrogen.

We are often told that these traits are simply genetic, but I personally whilst not being judgmental to the person, certainly raise an eyebrow and seriously question these claims. I discuss later about BPA in plastics and their oestrogen hormone mimicking effects in humans.

Cows are also administered routine antibiotics as a preventative measure against disease to compensate for the unhygienic, unnatural abhorrent conditions they have to endure within controlled animal feeding operations (CAFO's). Many poor beasts go through chronic pain and suffering with digestive diseases and infections and particularly mastitis. The routine antibiotics, growth hormones and steroids extend through into our food chain with the consumption of milk and the animals flesh.

It may not be just our medical institutes over prescription and use of antibiotics that are causing our immunity to antibiotics. Seventy percent of antibiotics that are manufactured go into our livestock industries in the feed and medically administered by injection. So, are you beginning to see the picture here? Animals routinely administered antibiotics within their feed and other routine disease preventative health measures serves as a major contributor to our overall immunity/resistance to antibiotics when it comes the time that we actually need them.

Antibiotics also serve to destroy the effectiveness of our digestive system and that of the animals by indiscriminately killing off 'all bacteria', both good and bad within our digestive tracts, inhibiting the body's absorbsion and assimilation of nutrients.

It should be understood that the digestive system makes up approximately eighty percent of our immune system and that by depleting the ecological balance of bacteria (good gut flora) undermines the body's overall ability to fight infection and disease and to assimilate nutrients from our food. If you are using a course of antibiotics it would be good practice to consume regular sources of pro-biotics and pre-biotics to replenish the good bacteria that the antibiotics destroy. Biotic means 'life' so understand that antibiotic means anti - life. On the other hand Probiotic means 'for life' to build life, to support life.

From my studies I understand that seventy percent of people whether they are aware of it or not have an allergy or intolerance to dairy products which may build up progressively.

People may just struggle to break down milk, placing stress on the body's digestive resources. Many people have varying degrees of undiagnosed allergic reactions to dairy products that they just live with, including; runny eyes, sinus and mucus problems, irritable bowel syndrome, digestive system inflammation, itchy scalp, eczema or psoriasis etc. Many of these issues are the body's natural reaction to rid itself of various toxins and unnatural foods.

If you visit the doctor for a food intolerance issue, the top two foods which trigger allergies or intolerances are, you guessed it, No. 1 Milk (dairy products) No. 2 Wheat and gluten intolerance. They are commonly known to cause the body to attack and turn on itself which is termed as an 'auto immune disease'.

The body will place toxins as far away from vital organs as it can. The toxins will end up being placed in fat, soft tissue, joints and ligaments, spots and acne. Anti-body's will then be sent out to attack the toxins and in doing so will attack joints creating inflammation (arthritis, tennis elbow), skin (Eczema, Psoriasis rosacea).

It might be an interesting idea to try a thirty-day "dairy fast," avoiding all dairy products and then monitor your symptoms and how you feel. I read that many people experience increased energy levels, and improved digestion and they typically see a strong improvement in mucus sinus conditions, asthma and eczema.

Milk and its contaminants have the potential to aggravate numerous common health issues in people and many people have not lived one single day without consuming processed cow's milk and dairy products. Most people are unaware of the possibility of a connection with their health conditions. Go on try it, just for thirty days without dairy and see for yourself how you feel.

My wife's friend had been going through intolerable hot flushes and night sweats for months which she presumed to be what is commonly referred to as, the Change. She cut out milk and dairy and the night sweats and hot flushes completely stopped after about a week of cutting out dairy.

We are now firmly of the opinion that things do not just happen without a reason and there are usually reasons for all of our ills. Cow's milk fed to babies according to various research sources is potentially highly damaging and may set the young person up for a lifetime of ills.

According to the World Health Organisation, in the first weeks in the life of a baby, the intestinal wall is extremely permeable, which allows foreign protein from cow's milk or formula to pass through into the blood stream in an undigested form. This can often set up the conditions for a lifetime of allergies and related syndromes, including milk-induced colitis and even sudden infant death from allergic reactions to cow's milk.

Studies have observed that on a diet high in casein (milk protein), the major source being dairy, some forms of cancer grew five times as fast.

The prestigious journal "Science" reported that based on a large body of evidence now available, there is in fact NO relationship between calcium intake and bone density. In fact dairy products exacerbate the problem, in that dairy is naturally high in protein and galactose milk sugar and actually promotes osteoporosis. The amino acids in milk protein increases blood acidity and the body draws calcium from the bones to neutralize this acidity. Greater amounts of calcium are therefore excreted in the urine. In Support of this protein osteoporosis connection, a University of Florida study found that vegetarian women had greater bone density and less calcium excretion than omnivores.

"Consumption of dairy products, particularly at age 20 years, was associated with an increased risk of hip fracture in old age. ("Case-Control Study of Risk Factors for Hip Fractures in the Elderly". American Journal of Epidemiology. Vol. 139, No. 5, 1994).

This seems to be indicating that Milk and other acidifying foods contribute to osteoporosis and brittle bones? We are all instilled with the notion that there is nothing on earth better for our bones than milk. Is all we have been bought up to know about the goodness of milk now been shattered as misconceptions or lies?

I am now led to believe that the process of milk pasteurization came into being not merely as an attempt to protect against harmful bacteria, allegedly found in raw milk. It may be likely from the need of large dairy corporations to increase shelf-life and the distance milk could be delivered before spoiling, hence increasing profits. Super-heated pasteurisation processes we are told kills off the bad bacteria, but nothing seems to be mentioned about it also killing off the beneficial bacteria and nutrients. Remember our body's need an ecological balance of bacteria for digestive functionality and maintaining an effective immune system.

Mass farmed cattle in 'confined animal feeding operations' (CAFO's) are now fed genetically modified corn based products as it is cheaper and serves to bulk up the cattle quickly.

These poor beasts never see the light of day, living unnatural miserable lives. Cows were never designed to eat corn! Where I come from cows were created to be outside in a field, with fresh air sunlight and eating grass. Where do you think cows get their large and tremendously strong bones from originally? That's right chlorophyll and calcium rich 'green grass with all its cofactors.

The stress placed on cows being factory farmed, not seeing the light of day, having its offspring dragged away, fed an unnatural diet is immense. This unnatural diet creates an unbalanced digestive ecology of gut flora that may have many far reaching health implications. Health issues like e-coli, helicobacter virus, salmonella, swine flu, bird flu etc. etc. are brandished by the health authorities and their health & safety scare mongering tactics through media in society.

I grew up on a farm and hey, I am still alive today having been faced with more muck than I care to remember and we were never constantly washing our hands with antibacterial soaps and solutions.

I believe things have dramatically changed by our modern corporate farming strategies to the detriment of the livestock and the consumer. Who knows the full implications of genetically modified corn used in animal feed and humanity!!! I believe that we are beginning to find out though as our health services spiral out of control to the crippling demand of our disease, sickness and stress related ailments.

The homogenisation process disperses the fat content of milk preventing it from separating out and floating to the top. This high pressure high heat process alters the chemistry of the milk fat on a molecular level, making it difficult for our digestive system to recognise and digest. Homogenization is an intense process that forcefully breaks up the fat molecules present in butterfat thus allowing them to be suspended in, rather than separated from the liquid milk itself. This intensive process leaves these delicate fats subject to oxidization. Oxidized fats contribute to heart disease, hypertension and hyperlipidemia (fats in the blood). The broken up unnatural fats are much smaller molecules and are able to enter into the blood stream in an undigested form which sets off the immune system attack and all sorts of auto immune responses.

We are led to believe that we need the calcium from milk, but we do not seem to be told that we can get all the calcium we need from eating green leafy vegetables and salads. Yes, simple greens!

It should be understood that to metabolise calcium into the bones there are essential co-factors that are important for bone health which are vitamin D, magnesium, boron, silica and very importantly vitamin k.

Without sufficient cofactors, assimilating calcium into our body is inhibited greatly and the calcium may be displaced in soft tissues and cause other issues like painful gall stones or kidney stones, bone spurs, arthritis and calcification in organs and cancer.

Oils, Fats and Spreads

Margarine,

Our continuing research led us to the conclusion that we should eliminate margarine from our diet as it contains unhealthy unnatural fats. Trans-fats, or hydrogenated fats are chemically altered vegetable oils that are not fully digestible by the human digestive system. I found that margarines are actually one molecule away from being plastic. They are produced artificially in a process called hydrogenation which turns liquid oil into solid fat at room temperature, of course for the consumer's convenience.

Margarine can be found in thousands of processed foods, from sweets, biscuits, cakes, cereals, pies and pastries to ready meals. They are used because they are cheap, add bulk to products, have no flavour and give products a longer shelf life. They have very little nutritional value.

I understand that there is much evidence to support that trans-fats and processed margarines build up within the body over time and clog up the arteries like a plaque, causing heart disease and cardio vascular problems when consumed regularly.

> "People are fed by the food industry which pays no attention to health and then treated by the health industry which pays no attention to food"
>
> **Wendell Berry**

Organic natural butter, in moderate amounts would be better than hydrogenated margarine even though the margarine is claiming to be low in fat and low cholesterol. Man's manipulating and bioengineering was enough for us to make our decision to remove margarine from our diet.

The Healthier Oils

Extra virgin olive oil, flax seed oil, or raw organic virgin coconut oil, are all healthier alternatives to traditional supermarket vegetable cooking oils.

We removed all commonly available processed vegetable cooking oil products and all partially-hydrogenated trans-fats that are known carcinogens (cancer causing) when continually heated or heated with high temperatures. We found that it was not advisable to heat any oil to excessive temperatures during cooking as this could cause acrylamide toxicity with cancer causing implications. Frying foods like the big English breakfast is generally speaking not the healthiest way of cooking but lightly stir frying vegetables we felt was acceptable to us using the healthier 'natural oils' and never using extreme temperatures with any oil. Organic Virgin rapeseed oil and virgin coconut oil were oils that apparently do stand up to higher temperatures.

Fatty products

Cancer sufferers should consider as we did the removal of all: pastries, cakes, pies, pasties, fried battered fish, chips, waffles, crisps, etc. This is also common sense for anyone to remove or reduce their intake of these dead foods.

I can already hear people complaining and bargaining with their lives, saying I would prefer to die happy eating all the foods I love to eat than to give them up. This is of course the individual's prerogative.

Supplementation

Additionally we supplemented our new improved diet by introducing vitamins, minerals and digestive enzymes & oils.

Vitamin C

Vitamin C (ascorbic acid) serves to oxygenate the body and is well reputed to have cancer inhibiting properties. When vitamin C is introduced into the body intravenously it creates hydrogen peroxide which oxygenates the cells and I understand is selectively cytotoxic to cancer cells. Glucose and vitamin C (ascorbate) have a very similar chemical makeup so could it be that this tricks the cancer cells into consuming the ascorbic acid thinking it to be sugar?

Vitamin C is water soluble and is very difficult to overdose on as it will simply be excreted within the urine. The worse that could happen realistically is that you reach bowel tolerance and it makes you have loose stools. If this happens reduce the amount to suit the individual.

Care is required in selecting good quality vitamin supplements as the cheap synthetic versions with all the bulking and caking agents and artificial flavours and sugars etc. may have health issues in themselves. Vitamin C also deals with mopping up free radicals which if allowed to go unchecked are known to encourage inflammation and cancer.

The great biochemist Linus Pauling, promoted orthomolecular (nutritional) medicine, megavitamin therapy, dietary supplements and also taking mega doses of vitamin C, especially with cancer. Pauling was the only person to receive two unshared Nobel Prize's one in chemistry and one as a peace activist, so this was a man of some standing. However as soon as he started to get involved in the cancer business and to tell the truth he found himself holding a 10,000 volt wire. Even though his life's work was amazing, he has been discredited on the drug funded 'quack watch' type websites who are in the pockets of the pharmaceutical corporations.

Digestive enzymes

Digestive enzymes help to support the body's own digestive system to break down nutrients from our foods. Our pancreas has to work hard to produce these enzymes to break down the nutrients from our food, especially when we do not eat foods that naturally contain their own live enzymes.

The pancreas and digestive system can be supported by introducing broad spectrum digestive enzyme supplementation, fermented foods, organic vegetables and salads that somehow seem so unpopular within today's younger society, particularly with children.

There are whole cancer protocols surrounding the power of particularly proteolytic enzymes and their ability to break down the fibrin coating surrounding the cancer cells. The fibrin has a negative charge attached to it which buffers against the negative charge of our immune cells. This is like placing to magnets together of the same polarity, they repel. If the coating is removed then our white blood cells, T lymphocytes can draw up to the cancer and see that there is something not right and draw to arms.

Multi Vitamin

We used a good multi vitamin for a general all round supplementation.

Vitamin D3 (AKA sunshine)

Vitamin D3 is also known to be an excellent anti-cancer vitamin and all round vital immune system booster. Vitamin D is oil soluble and in fact is not a vitamin but is a steroidal hormone. The majority of cancer patients when tested will find that they are vitamin D deficient. This vitamin is essential to human health and we get the majority through our skins exposure to sunlight which is manufactured in a synthesis with the sun's rays and cholesterol under our skin. Yet we are told don't go out into the sun as it causes cancer!!!?

Try researching the chemicals used within sun cream and this will really open your eyes as to the real 'factors', forgive the pun! Enter in the name of the individual chemical in the sun cream followed by MSDS and read through the 'material safety data sheet' to open up a disturbing reality. Many contain Benzene or Benzene related chemicals which are carcinogenic especially when heated! Sun = Sunscreen = heat = toxin release = potential carcinogenic reactions within the skin.

Vitamin D can be bought in supplement form, spray form or simply having skin exposure to sunshine as the most natural way. Without vitamin D3, Vitamin K2 and Magnesium the body is unable to process and utilise calcium from the foods we eat, potentially leading to osteoarthritis (brittle bones). The truth is you do not have to remember all of these complexities just eat plenty of raw greens and colour of the rainbow fruits and vegetables and enjoy the beautiful sunshine.

Acidophilus,

This is a Probiotic we used to build up the good bacteria within the gut intestines and to thereby build the overall immune system and digestion as eighty percent of the immune system is within the gut. A healthy gut also has a direct effect on mood and cognitive function. How we feel in our mind and emotions are all factors in our holistic health

Exercise,

Exercise serves to enrich the body with cancer inhibiting oxygen directly into the cells and it also releases endorphins which make you feel great. Exercise is also a good form of de-stressing and assists in maintaining a flowing lymphatic system which is the sewage system for getting rid of cellular waste and toxicity.

With our modern sedentary lifestyles we need to move more in order to prevent our lymphatic system from stagnating and toxic build up. Our blood or vascular system has a pump (the heart) but the lymphatic system does not and it relies on the movement, contraction and expansion of our muscles for it to displace the waste toxins from cells into the liver and then out of the body.

An excellent way of getting the lymphatic system moving is by the use of a 'rebounder' which is a small exercise trampoline. You do not even have to be bouncing as high as Tigger from Winnie the Poo either, so don't worry. You can just gently balance which will provide muscle contraction and expansion moving the lymphatic fluid and getting toxins moving out. You can then just build on this, in whatever you can achieve.

According to Ciaran Devane, chief executive of Macmillan Cancer Support,

"Cancer patients would be shocked if they knew just how much of a benefit physical activity could have on their recovery and long term health, in some cases reducing their chances of having to go through the grueling ordeal of treatment all over again..."

Hyperbaric Oxygen Therapy

There is another way of oxygenating the body which could potentially be a very important part of the cancer fighting armory; this is Hyperbaric Oxygen Therapy (HBO).

HBO is a process whereby the body is placed in a chamber which is pressurized and you breath pure 100% medical grade oxygen. The system is just like going into an aeroplane pressurized environment. This allows enriched oxygen to be taken deep into the cells of the body and creates a healthy oxygen saturated body which is an unfriendly environment for cancer cells. This is particularly effective when on the ketogenic diet. Sue did not do HBO simply because we were unaware of the benefits at the time.

The HBO is also highly effective in healing scar tissue caused through medical standard of care treatments i.e. radiation burns, surgery, and chemotherapy tissue damage. Not only is the HBO effective in healing scar tissue but it is also extremely effective in getting enriched oxygen directly into the cancer cells.

(Brizel DM et al; The mechanisms by which oxygen and carbogen improve tumour oxygenation - Br J Cancer 1995; 72; 1120-1124)

When looking for a HBO center try to find an MS charity organization as opposed to privately run because the costs can vary significantly. We have a local MS center in Nottingham which charges a £20.00 yearly membership fee and then £12.00 per hours session. We have heard of private HBO centers charging up to £250 per hour.

Colonics

Cleansing the Colon may not be the most popular topics of conversation, but we firmly believe this to be a vitally important health protocol. With the build-up of toxicity from modern day foods and lifestyle it is so important to create an efficient eliminatory system to get those toxins out as soon as you can.

It is quite unsettling to realise that there is a debris of toxic waste clinging to the insides of your large intestines/bowels. This mucus plaque like build up continues to leach bacteria from putrefying waste material back into the body causing a continuous long term exposure to toxins within the body and a constant strain on the immune system.

The colon cleanse therefore was to clean out the pipes so to speak, disabling this source of stagnating toxicity and enabling toxins from deeper within the body to be eliminated efficiently.

We used a colon cleanse called Colonics which consisted largely of Magnesium Oxide which works by hydrating the bowels giving a thorough but gentle cleanse. We purchased this from Phillip Day of Credence within the UK: www.credenceonline.co.uk. This is where we also purchased our Hunza bitter apricot kernels. Of course there may be many other good sources of colon cleanse, but we trusted Phillip Day as he is one of the good guys.

We drank plenty of fresh pure water whilst doing the colon cleanse as this works in unison with the colonics powder by hydration and loosening the plaque. Sue took half a teaspoon of the colonics powder mixed in a glass of warm water every morning for ten days.

The colon cleanse was important for us to do prior to the liver cleanse in order to create an efficient eliminatory system.

With most people this cleanse is quite gentle does not cause a running to the toilet all day long. However, everyone is different and there has been one or two people at our meetings who have mentioned "do you know that colonics you mentioned"!!! Just follow the recommendations of the manufacturer or your healthcare professional and if you find that it is shall we say 'over stimulating' then simply cut back a little on the dosage.

We always recommend that people seek guidance from a professional nutritionist or healthcare professional especially in the case of a poorly functioning liver. Toxins contained in the body could overload a poorly functioning liver when coming out which is why professional guidance may be required.

Please do not get the colon cleanse confused with an enema as they are not the same so you can now breathe a sigh of relief.

We did not do enemas, but I understand that enemas are an excellent additional part of the detoxification and cancer fighting armoury. Enemas serve to efficiently clean out the bowels and coffee enemas in particular stimulate the liver into overdrive and enable efficient removal of toxicity from the liver. This is particularly important when doing lots of juicing, i.e. Gerson therapy

Therefore coffee enemas are a very good thing as usually most people who have cancer contain a lot of toxicity within their body which needs to come out as part of their healing. Many toxins are contained within the fat cells, so when people juice, come off the carbs and sugars they start losing fat cells which releases the toxins into the body which can overload the liver.

When tumour cells start breaking down too, where do you think they go to be removed from the body, you guessed it poor old liver. We also used the herb Milk Thistle which can be helpful in greatly supporting the liver.

Good or not so good?

Bread, is it good for us?

We decided to take white bread out of our diet as research showed quite conclusively that it has no appreciable nutritional value. White flour goes through refining processes which takes out the wheat germ nutrient and bran fibre which renders it nutritionally depleted. It may also be bleached using chemical bleaching agents, Chlorine (oxidiser) Hydrochloric Acid (reducing agent) to make white and more visually appealing bread. It is then dried in kilns at high temperature which kill any remaining beneficial nutrients. My understanding is that white bread can be likened to eating cardboard as it is so devoid of nutrition.

White bread is not only lacking in nutrient content but it actually inhibits the body's ability to take in nutrients from other foods as the sticky dough paste 'glu - ten' coats the nutrient absorbing nodules (Villi) within the small intestines, inhibiting the absorbsion of nutrients from other foods passing through. This information is important to everyone but particularly people who have cancer as up to 40% of cancer patients suffer from malnutrition or cachexia which is a complex malabsorption and recycling of energy issue where the cancer feeds itself and muscle wasting ensues.

One major cause of the body's inability to absorb nutrients can be chemotherapy which destroys fast growing cells in the body, i.e. cancer cells. The problem is that there are many other fast growing cells within the body, namely hair, nails, the stomach lining and mucus membranes throughout the digestive system, throat and mouth. Therefore we need to optimise nutritional uptake, not inhibit it. Unfortunately this sort of information is not explained by oncologists as they have no training in nutrition.

Their answer seems to be to recommend high sugar and processed fatty products including: cakes, biscuits, puddings, milk and dairy, along with sugary drinks etc. etc. to prevent losing weight. These are not what I would consider healthy recommendations or convalescence foods. What good would high calorie sugar intake have in creating a healthy body and supporting the immune system? These calories (units of energy) will usually serve to feed the cancer (glycolysis) or be converted to fat and will put weight on, but what good is fat when muscle mass is being wasted through malabsorption of nutrients. I think that the cancer industry does not want it publicized that 40% of cancer patients die through starvation /cachexia which may be exacerbated by their treatments. What is their answer, keep the weight on at all costs, even if that is going to feed the cancer starches, glucose & sugars, the very thing cancer needs to thrive.

Something also to be aware of is that some brown bread may be actually white bread that has been dyed using brown caramel dye (E150). I understand that there are studies to suggest that this E150 brown dye is implicated in gastro-intestinal allergic reactions in sensitive people. This brown bread is a deception and is not the same as 'wholemeal' brown bread it just looks the part.

We made the decision to limit the consumption of bread mainly due to the starch content that turns immediately to sugar and strong evidence supporting that particularly processed sugar is oncogenic and feeds cancer. This is where we used moderation but chose wisely which type of bread. We did eat small quantities of wholemeal bread as well as some of the ancient grained bread.

The breads that we considered including in our diet were breads where the grain had not undergone genetic modification or extensive corporate agricultural farming and processing. These ancient grains used in breads include; Millet, Rye, Spelt, Barley which were in our view not perfect but better choices than brown dye bread, wholemeal or white bread.

Flat breads or heavy dense breads baked without the use of synthetic yeast are also a healthier choice. There are also sour dough fermented breads, which have a good live bacterial culture which helps break down allergenic gluten and assists in the body's digestive processes.

Another issue with wheat from corporate agriculture is that when the time comes for harvest the wheat is sprayed with glyphosate (highly toxic herbicide) which poisons the wheat plant. However, in the plants last death throws to survive it releases its seeds more readily which makes harvesting much more efficient and cost effective and ultimately more profitable. The only down side to this is that it is now toxic to humans in long term consumption and to some in the shorter term like celiac disease, IBS or people suffering numerous undiagnosed digestive disorders. We now understand that bread and wheat in general are not the best choices of food when people have cancer or not.

- According to The World Health Organization (WHO), Glyphosate is classed as a category 2a carcinogen, which means the it is a probable cause of cancer

- The beneficial good gut bacteria are directly in the path of harm caused by glyphosate's toxic mechanism. Our intestinal microbes have the same pathway used by glyphosate to kill weeds.

- Glyphosate causes extreme disruption of microbes' functions and lifecycles. What is more concerning is that glyphosate preferentially damages beneficial bacteria within our gut, allowing pathogens to multiply out of control.

Food preservatives

We decided to remove foods containing unnatural and what we considered harmful preservatives. Preservatives are additives placed into foods to prolong shelf life and keep the products from being spoiled or broken down by micro-organisms. Such preservatives include; Sulphites, BHT & BHA, refined sugar, Sodium Nitrate and Nitrite, Brominated Vegetable oil (BVO) sulphur dioxide, to name but a few. These are contained in many foods like Ham, smoked foods, salted products, tinned products, industry produced jams, processed oils, margarines, pickled products, etc. Basically most things that would normally go off in natural circumstances but last months if not years with preservatives added. I refer back to one of my common sayings: "if the bugs or bacteria do not want to eat it, then why would we?"

We removed all processed/re-constituted foods, i.e. sausages, burgers, sausage rolls, scampi, chicken nuggets, etc. This is highly acidifying food, unhealthy fats using mulched animal waste products, loaded with taste enhancing MSG, colorants and flavourings with little nourishment. But don't kids just love them though!!!

Sugar

Sue took out ALL refined sugars, artificial sugars/sweeteners and natural foods with high starch/sugars i.e. certain fruits and some root vegetables. Whilst fruit is great (skins and all), our understanding was that the high glycaemic fruits do represent an issue in people who have cancer, as all sugars serve to fuel cancer cells. Juicing fruits can spike blood sugar levels through taking out the fibre which normally slows the absorbsion of sugars into the blood.

The University of California states that thirty five million people die each year of sugar related health issues, whilst 7.5 million die from alcohol and smoking related health issues.

Our decision was that Sue as a Cancer sufferer may have apples and pears if not too over ripe and lemons and limes. Water melon can also be a wonderfully rich source of nutrients, minerals and hydration. Chewing the pips/seeds, can also be highly nutritious from these low glycaemic fruits. We also included Pineapples because we understood that they were helpful as they contained Bromelain which is a powerful proteolytic enzyme (digests Proteins) and natural anti-cancer agent especially when taken to work synergistically with Vitamin B17 (apricot kernels).

Salt

Table salt is a refined processed product made from two toxic components, sodium and chloride, with no health benefits and is detrimental to health used in excess. If a salt is pure white and says it is sea salt then bear in mind that there is a reason for its pure whiteness and that reason is; man's processing!

However, unprocessed natural salt can be highly beneficial to health as it contains seventy plus minerals in balance with the sodium and chloride. The type of salt I am referring to is the highly mineralised natural sea salt. We threw out the processed table salt and replaced this with 'Celtic sea salt' or 'grey salt', containing many minerals which are very important in the functioning of a healthy body. We also use pink Himalayan Rock salt which is wonderfully mineralised and alkalising. However, whilst this is natural and healthier than processed salt, we chose to use this in moderation as we did not want to over load on sodium.

Shell fish

Shellfish are basically ocean floor scavengers which serve to clean up the decaying putrefying debris from the sea bed. We removed most shellfish/crustaceans from our diet due to well documented toxicity levels inherent to the type of species that they are. Many of these creatures are known to contain high levels of toxicity including mercury. I have to admit that we struggled to give up seafood, especially prawns being one of our favourites.

Herbs and Spices

Rosemary, thyme, oregano, basil, mint, fresh nettle tea, Cumin, turmeric, cinnamon, coriander, Ginger plus many other herbs and spices are amazing nutrients for the body. These are great for your immune system and Turmeric is widely known even in medical studies to have incredible anti-cancer and anti-inflammatory properties. I enjoy making a winter warmer tea out of Turmeric, Cayenne pepper, Ginger, Star Anise and Cloves with a little local raw honey (not processed) to sort out cold and flu symptoms.

Of course if you have cancer you may want to moderate the honey content due to the sugar feeds cancer issue. Sometimes however utilising raw honey or natural molasses in conjunction with anti-cancer herbs, foods or supplements we understood could assist in there penetration into the cancer cell structure. This is where perhaps the saying comes from "a spoon full of sugar helps the medicine go down" not only taste wise but opening up the cancers glucose receptors to take up cancer fighting nutrients in conjunction with the honey/sugar.

Cancer desperately seeks sugar as fuel, and like a Trojan horse the sugar takes with it anti-cancer Turmeric, vitamin B17, or vitamin C straight to the cancer cells. Consult your holistic health care practitioner further about these protocols.

Drinks

We invested in a water filter and drank at least one and a half litres to two litres of pure water each day. This is a vital part of flushing out the body and detoxification. It is important not to drink too much water when you are having a meal as this serves to dilute the digestive enzymes and Hydrochloric acid within the stomach which would inhibit digestion. Cold water when taken with meals will also diminish the enzyme activity within the stomach which are needed to efficiently break down food.

We removed black tea and coffee (caffeine products) and we did not resort to decaffeinated either as this goes through man's chemical treatment processes to extract the caffeine. We removed cartons of preserved fruit juices, absolutely no highly acidifying energy or fizzy sugary drinks, no artificial flavoured or sweetened dilute juice. Much of the supermarket dilute juice contains artificial sweeteners like Aspartame which goes under the guise of many other artificial sugar names ending in ----cose, ---lose, or ----tose. If you notice the common theme here it is all referring to highly processed foods and drinks isn't it?

We introduced green teas and herbal teas, many of which Sue began to grow fresh in our own garden which are great anti-oxidants and antioxidants are well renowned to help prevent cancer and chronic disease. Sue's favourites were Rosemary and Oregano which she says are an acquired taste but they were part of the cancer fighting armoury, being packed full of super goodness. I too love the oregano tea in particular.

Green tea still contains caffeine but the benefits of the anti-oxidants are amazing and are well worth having. Other herbal teas we used were; Mint, Ginger, lemon balm, nettle, dandelion, sprinkling in variations of turmeric, cinnamon, Star anise, Cayenne pepper to taste. I chose a little local unprocessed honey, but Sue refrained from sweet things.

We did buy in small amounts of Goats milk which we understood to be a healthier alternative to cow's milk as it is more similar to human milk and our body is able to digest it far easier. However whilst I used this sue stuck to rice milk, almond milk and coconut milk. The nut milks we made by using a blender and blending the nuts with water and then straining through a cheese or muslin cloth, a surprisingly wonderful alternative to animal milk.

Microwave cooking

Although very convenient, I understood that microwave cooking was unnatural and denatures nutrients and destroys natural enzymes in our food. The radiation microwaves change the food on a molecular level creating a product that the body does not easily recognise to digest and assimilate into the body. As previously mentioned I read that the body develops white blood cell activity to fight against denatured unnatural food in a process called 'Digestive Leuko cytosis'. I discovered that the microwave was invented by the Nazi's in world war two in order to feed their field troops. This technology was then taken and developed by the Russians who subsequently banned its use in 1976 due to its health implications but the west ran with it. I find it interesting that Russia banned use of the microwave in 1976 and they also banned genetically modified crops in contrast to our western government's embracement.

Microwave cooking often uses plastic containers in ready meals etc. which release xenoestrogens from the plastics, which are female hormone mimickers. Bisphenol A. (BPA) is the hardening compound used in the plastics industry which is released from the plastic into foods through heat, time and acidity. These types of plasticisers may be hormonally disruptive within our body.

Hormone mimicking plastics

Heating food in plastics or wrapped with cellophane or exposing plastics to sunlight is known to release bisphenol A (BPA). BPA is known to induce Xenoestrogens which are implicated in cancer due to their hormone disrupting roll and the development or feeding of reproductive system cancers. Although we know that many of the reproductive organ cancers are oestrogen driven, we keep loading our bodies with

> Release of Bisphenol A is exacerbated through;
>
> Heat, Time and Acidity

this toxic onslaught of artificial hormones and the doctors prescribe hormone blocking drugs as opposed to advising people against ingesting synthetic sources of these hormones. The general public remain unquestioningly unaware.

The simple thing to remember in this is, wherever practical refrain from using plastics in the storage or preparation of food and drink, especially if heating it up, extended storage duration and acidic foods which leach the BPA more readily.

Question, why don't the innocent looking tea bags disintegrate like normal paper when water is poured over them as surely they are only paper aren't they? The reason is that the paper is plasticised and we pour boiling water on the plasticised bag releasing plasticiser chemicals within the tea. The same companies that make teabags also make cigarette papers and for the same reason why do the papers not break down with the moistness of your saliva? Go to the top of the class, yes it is plasticised, the same paper as receipts from supermarkets.

Why do cats find it irresistible to spray or mark their territory over plastic bags, tents, builders plastic etc.? They sense the hormone characteristics within the plastic.

In our Western industrialized society we are progressively exposed to more and more xenoestrogen hormone mimickers.

These plastics are prevalent in modern society through our environment, via pesticides, herbicides, fungicides, plastics, perfume, H&B products, fuels, car exhausts, dry cleaning chemicals, industrial waste, meat from animals which have been fattened with estrogenic drugs, and countless other household and personal products which many of us use every day. This is another reason to go organic and all natural.

Other Influencing Factors.

I continue to reiterate that we should be looking to eat foods which are fresh and as close to their natural state as possible. This is if we are looking for a healthier life, or redressing the effects of a lifetime of unhealthy eating and lifestyle. There are other factors such as personal care and hygiene products and household cleaning products that are potentially damaging to health such as shampoos, talcum powder, deodorants, household bleach, air fresheners, anti-bactericidal cleaning agents, soaps and fluoride in toothpaste.

Yes, toothpaste, which contains sodium fluoride which is one of the main constituents in rat poison. If you read on the side of the tube it states that if a child swallows a pea sized amount then you should get them checked out by a doctor. There is of course naturally occurring calcium fluoride in minimal quantities found in nature which is what people often argue is good for us. Then there is hydro fluorosilicic acid, which is the fluoride placed in our municipal water supply that comes from the chemical smelting process of the aluminium industry and the phosphate mining industry. This fluoride is a toxic waste bi-product which is used in our water supplies.

It is interesting to note that the toxic waste is shipped in tankers from China stated as a water treatment but it is also specified as a very potent pesticide/insecticide.

There is much controversy over its use to fluoridate our water supplies. I read that the Nazi party used fluoride to dull down the Jews and prevent them from breeding, that's was a real shocker to me! Even if there was merit in the use of fluoride from this toxic waste bi product for dental integrity, purely from a business perspective it seems illogical to waste that entire product in the water supply when we only actually physically consume about three percent of the water that comes through the tap. The other ninety seven percent goes on washing your clothes, car, windows, watering the garden, bathing, showering fish tank etc.

What a tremendous waste of product if fluoride is placed in our total water supplies for dental reasons only. This seems to me to be a slow build up toxicity that our bodies would do well not to have. Sue and I also sourced fluoride free toothpaste. We also made up all-natural toothpaste using organic virgin coconut oil mixed with bicarbonate of soda and a few drops of peppermint oil which is amazing.

There are also health issues that are sometimes more of a challenge to overcome in modern society, like radiation contamination, telephone masts, mobile phones, radio frequency waves, electromagnetic wiring in households etc. etc.

Electromagnetics

We removed electrical wiring from our sleeping area at night. Even if the electrical wire is not being used by an appliance there is still electricity in the wire and this gives out electromagnetic forces which can build up within areas where you may be laid asleep for eight hours at a time, night after night.

Consider getting a battery alarm clock or moving the electric alarm further away from the bed area.

You may wish to refrain from smart meters being installed and wifi. Maybe hardwire directly to the modem system to restrict radio frequency wave contamination that is often implicated in cancer and brain tumours. Excessive use of mobile phones may also be something to look into and maybe use the speaker phone to keep the phone away from the head. Keep conversations short on any home cordless phone or mobile phone and consider hard wired land line phones.

Bathing and showering

We wash, shower or bathe day in day out, without giving to much thought to what we are allowing to penetrate our bodies. Our skin is the largest organ of our body which is permeable. It is worth understanding that what is present in the water, has direct access into the metropolis of our body through skin absorbsion.

Chemicals like chlorine, fluoride, bactericides in soaps and detergents, foaming chemicals like sodium laureth and sodium lauryl sulphate, perfume chemicals and hormone disrupting petrochemicals from H & B products. All of these toxins are readily absorbed into the bloodstream through our skin. The hotter the water, the more readily it opens up the skins pores giving direct access into the blood stream.

> ### Healthy philosophy
>
> If you wouldn't eat it then don't put it on your skin!

Using soaps and shampoo's over the whole of the body breaks down the surface tension of the skin and the body's natural protective oils allowing total 'access granted' to chemical penetration breaching through our body's first line of defence.

Chlorine and fluoride are also toxic chemicals that are contained in many of our mains water supply networks. When they are continually entering into our body day after day, week after week and year after year this progressively takes its toll, placing toxic stresses on your body.

Soaps, shampoos and toothpaste usually contain chemicals such as Sodium Laureth Sulphate and Lauryl Sulphate which give them there foaming action. These chemicals are also used in engine de-greasants. Consider restricting soap and shampoo's to be used predominantly under the arms and in the groin areas. Try to obtain more natural products with less perfume additives which can often be endocrine disrupters, creating hormonal imbalance.

The body produces an oily substance in the skin called sebum which serves as a natural protective barrier and has water resistance qualities. Soaps and detergents wash away the sebum and allow impurities and chemicals to enter in through the skin and get into the bloodstream more readily. The removal of the sebum also has health implications in terms of its use in metabolisation and manufacture of vitamin D from the sunlight.

The manufacturing of vitamin D3 within the skin takes a couple of days, so when you shower using hot water and detergent shampoos over your whole body you are washing away the oils and the skins capacity in the production of vitamin D which is one of the most anti-cancer vitamins you could wish to have. Cancer patients in general have significantly low vitamin D levels.

In summary, try to refrain from bathing or showering using excessively hot water in conjunction with petrochemical derived soaps and detergents. Better still source and use natural non perfumed soap and shampoos using in minimal quantities as possible and concentrating their use under the arms and groin areas. Look to bathe in mineral rich salts which you may then increase the temperature in order to maximise the absorbsion of these health minerals through the skin. Consider getting a shower water filter.

Health & Beauty products

Chemical heavy metals like arsenic, cadmium, mercury, lead and aluminium are often contained in makeup and many health and beauty products which are highly toxic. There are studies that have been done by the Environmental Defence, Ontario, in Canada that are damning. They state figures of five pounds in weight of toxic makeup sludge being absorbed into a woman's body on average each year through make up use.

Environmental Defense tested 49 different face makeup items, including four concealers, five foundations, four powders, five bronzers or blushes, seven mascaras, two eye liners, 14 eye shadows, and eight lipsticks or glosses. Their testing revealed serious heavy metal contamination in virtually all of the products:

> "Heavy metals are in our face makeup, and consumers have no way of knowing about it"
>
> **ENVIRONMENTAL DEFENCE**
> **Ontario Canada**

- 96 percent contained lead
- 90 percent contained beryllium
- 61 percent contained thallium
- 51 percent contained cadmium
- 20 percent contained arsenic

When someone is going through cancer one part of the armoury is to limit exposure to toxicity from all sources to prevent the over burdening of the immune system.

Food & Drink Examples

Breakfast

Wake up to a fresh lemon drink using a freshly squeezed lemon. Organic unsweetened cereal (rye, muesli, porridge) with rice milk, coconut milk or nut milk with organic blueberries. Lightly buttered sour dough toast (fermented bread) or millet, spelt, amaranth bread with free range scrambled egg or gently fried egg using raw virgin coconut oil with fresh tomatoes and a small sprinkle of pink Himalayan rock salt

Green Juices throughout the day, with varieties of spinach, cabbage, Kale, celery, or cucumber and mixed with options of carrots, apple, pear or lemon for slight sweetness but low glycaemic (low sugar). Pineapples are also known to be good which contain the proteolytic enzyme bromelain. Studies I have read show the value of proteolytic enzymes in breaking down the fibrin protective shield that surrounds the cancer allowing the immune system to recognise and attack.

Raw vegetable juicing may not be everyone's favourite initially, but the green wonder juice is the closest thing to blood haemoglobin, but from plant source. Haemoglobin are the tiny molecules within the blood that serve to transport oxygen.

The body needs iron, vitamin B12 and folic acid to make haemoglobin from our food.

This mega nutritional blast of juicing gets straight into your blood stream as the fibre has been removed which normally slows the absorbsion process down. The nutrients are assimilated very efficiently and the health benefits from this cannot be over stated. Try to use organic or fresh responsibly farmed local produce and 'just do it'!!! To get the best and most flavoursome juices I would suggest looking into Jason Vale 'The Juice Master'.

When juicing, try to change around and vary the types of green leafy vegetables to prevent overloading on certain nutrients. For a couple of days have spinach and then change to chard, then kale. Don't worry too much about being hard and fast about this, just change things around a little and see this as adding variety and colour of the rainbow produce.

We were mindful not to juice too many fruits as this could serve to spike blood sugar levels causing a rush of insulin. We also did not want to feed the cancer sugar although there is a big difference between processed sugars and natural whole fruits containing their fibre to slow down the absorbsion of the natural fruit sugar.

When drinking the juice remember to first swill it around mouth before swallowing which will allow the amylase enzyme from the six saliva ducts in the mouth to start to break down the nutrients. This is the first port of the digestive process. Chew the juice!

Here is one of our favourite juice blends

One whole organic lemon (skin and all)
Half an organic cucumber
Two organic green apples
Chunk of ginger to taste
One beetroot
A handful of dark green kale

Possibly add celery to enrich this nutrient power house.

Juicing recipe number two

Handful of curly Kale,
Two carrots
Half a cucumber,
Half a broccoli (stalks and florets)
Half or a full lemon (skin and all)
An apple/pear for sweetness,
Piece of ginger.

Experiment with the ratios and have fun making your own concoctions. Enjoy!

Nut Milks It is amazing how easy nut milks are to make and they are so good for you. Nut milk is packed full of protein from plant source which is readily digestible. Nut milk helps to build up the muscles and are a source of good fats for energy in the absence of simple carbohydrates and sugars. The ketogenic diet focusses on replacing good fats in place of carbs and sugars for energy source thereby not feeding the cancer cells their prime energy source but giving the normal cells energy through good oils. It is also important to inhibit muscle wasting through cachexia which is common following chemotherapy treatments.

All that you need to make this beautiful milk is raw nuts (not peanuts) of your choice, water, a blender and a strainer or muslin cloth. Sue used cashews and almonds placing them in a blender with water, blend, then strain. You can use the milk as you would cow's milk and the left over nuts for baking.

Dinner: Whole meal brown rice or small jacket potato. Oily Fish or organic chicken, Broccoli, spinach, cabbage, kale or salads with bean sprouts etc. Fermented sauerkraut, grated beetroot, salad and garnish with fresh herbs, lemon juice and or apple cider vinegar..

Stir fry – Bean sprouts, red peppers, carrots chicken, spices turmeric, ginger, Cayenne pepper and plenty of fresh herbs etc.

Homemade curry: with Chicken, wholegrain rice or bulgar wheat and load in plenty of herbs & spices like turmeric, ginger, coconut and coconut milk, black pepper, onions, garlic, okra, coriander, cinnamon, star anise etc. What a power house of goodness and toxin chelates. Chelation is the act of a compound that binds to heavy metal toxins within the body and assists in their removal.

Immune boosting soup

- 250g or 9oz of sweet potato peeled and chopped
- 250g or 9oz of carrots scrubbed and chopped
- One medium sized butternut squash, peeled and chopped
- 350 ml or 12 fl oz of vegetable stock
- 100ml or 3.5 fl oz of coconut milk
- 2 cm or 1inch piece of ginger, chopped or grated
- One tea spoon of ground mixed spice
- Clove of garlic
- Teaspoon of turmeric

Boil all the vegetables for fifteen minutes, puree in a blender with the coconut milk and add pepper to taste.

Immune Boosting Salad

- Broad beans, broccoli (raw), grated carrot, grated beetroot (raw), courgettes, watercress, lettuce, tomatoes, avocado. Add seeds or nuts or both and dress with extra virgin olive oil or walnut oil containing some crushed garlic. Add fresh garden mint, squeezed lemon and or apple cider vinegar with mother.

A useful suggestion would be to purchase a good 'vegetarian' cook book which have many beautiful dishes and then pack them with extra herbs and spices to taste. You could also add in some good quality organically sourced chicken (white meat) or fish if that is your preference. Oily fish we considered very good especially for a rich source of omega 3 fatty acids and small extra source of vitamin D.

My wife initially found it challenging in trying to adjust to the new lifestyle and eating regime at first, but after practice and consulting a very helpful professional nutritionist, things became easier, clearer and more manageable.

Summary of Lifestyle Changes

Summary of the most important strategies and immediate changes we put into place when Sue was going through cancer.

Detoxification First

Cleanse the colon. People can have up to 3kg of toxic debris clinging to the inside of their bowel walls. This becomes a breeding ground for bacteria, parasites and all sorts of nasties which are then reabsorbed by the body through the bowel walls. Colonics serves to loosen accumulated mucus plaque debris and toxins from within the bowels, hydrates and cleanses allowing efficient elimination of toxicity debris and waste materials.

We used a very gentle product called 'Colonics' by Vital Minerals. The Magnesium Oxide salt powder is mixed in a glass of water and drunk every morning for ten days. It was our understanding that the colon cleanse should be the first protocol to do and prior to the liver cleanse. Most naturopaths would say that healing starts in the colon.

Liver Detoxification: Cleansing the liver was the second stage protocol which comprised blending; up to one third of a pineapple (including the stem), a two to three centimetre chunk of ginger, one clove of garlic, and a tablespoon full of extra virgin olive oil (or flaxseed oil). Add some filtered water to liquefy to a suitable consistency. We drank this every morning, thirty minutes before eating any other foods. Sue did this for ten days.

It was advisable to come off of caffeinated products three days prior to and during the liver detox program. It is also important to retain fibre in the diet during a detoxification to allow the toxins to bind to the fibre and prevent re-absorbsion of toxins back into the body. It is also worth noting that you may not feel well during detox as the liver is placed under the stress of dealing with all the toxins coming out. People may experience flu like symptoms, which is why maintaining good fibre levels are important and to support the liver with milk thistle. Care is also needed to prevent overdoing things which could serve to over burden the liver and a sign of over burdening and poisoning the liver is where the skin and eyes start to turn yellow. Sue did not enjoy this detox but knew that it was important. The liver can also benefit from the supplement milk thistle and also coffee enemas which greatly support the liver in getting the toxins removed efficiently.

Parasite Cleanse, Parasites come in all sizes from large to microscopic, but they all compromise the body and immune system. We used a tincture of wormwood, black walnut hull and cloves which we purchased from a local medical herbalist. We had a few drops in a glass of water and built up the dose gradually over a period of three weeks. Seek specific guidance from the source of the parasite cleanse.

We refrained from the following:

- All processed sugar and sugar rich foods and especially artificial sweeteners Aspartame (we were in no doubt that sugar served to feed cancer through glycolysis)

- No dairy products, although Sue allowed herself a little organic butter.

- No standard vegetable cooking oils and artificial transfats and hydrogenated fats (margarine)

- No processed foods, nothing in packaging with ingredient names we could not pronounce.

- No preserved foods, tinned foods.

- No Food colorants

- No white bread, white flour or white rice

- No simple carbohydrates which turn immediately to sugar

- No fizzy drinks, energy drinks or dilute fruit drinks

- No alcohol

- No coffee (minimize caffeine)

- No red meat as this requires massive amounts of the body's energy and enzyme resources. This depletes pancreatic enzymes which could be placed to better use in fighting cancer and building up the immune system.

- Reduce/remove starchy root vegetables which turn immediately to sugar, such as potatoes, turnips and especially parsnips. We did Juice beetroot and carrots in green leafy vegetable blends. We had small jacket potato

- Fruit contains natural sugar so we reduced their intake. However we included Pineapple which contains the proteolytic enzyme Bromelain, which we understood to have wonderful cancer fighting properties. Organic apples and pears, lemons & limes were also acceptable within green juices. We refrained from over ripe fruit as this has more sugar in it.

- We got rid of the processed table salt and changed it for Himalayan mineralized rock salt or Celtic Sea Salt used in moderation.

- No microwave

- If it had a label of ingredients we could not pronounce, we refrained from it.

Sues Body intake regime

- Supplement with digestive enzymes, acidophilus, Vitamin D3 with K2.

- Organic extra virgin (cold pressed) olive oil or flaxseed oil, organic virgin coconut oil, black seed oil.

- Vitamin C intake (look at Liposomal) Consider higher than the recommended daily allowance (RDA). We understood that it was actually difficult to overdose on vitamin C and the worse that would happen when you reach saturation point would be to cause loose stools. We could then reduce the amount to bowel tolerance.

- We felt Vitamin B17 apricot Kernels were a vital part of the armoury and Sue took five or six at a time throughout the day to a maximum of thirty to thirty five per day. These were chewed to a pulp before swallowing.

- We often used vitamin B3, Niacin when eating apricot kernels and supplements to allow deeper nutrient absorbsion into the body. Niacin serves to dilate the small blood vessels under the skin opening up these small capillary blood vessels which allows deeper accessibility for oxygenation, phytonutrients going in and toxicity coming out. Niacin causes a tingling red skin flush which was a little strange at first but passed after about twenty minutes.

- Juicing raw green leafy and cruciferous vegetables, cucumber, celery, beetroot, carrots and adding an apple, pear or carrot to sweeten and make more interesting & palatable. Ginger, lemons, limes, turmeric root.

- Eat cartloads of raw vegetables and salads sourced from local organic or responsibly farmed outlets. (We ceased to place our trust in supermarket produce)

- Eat plenty of green leafy vegetables, like spinach, Kale, broccoli, cabbage and other cruciferous vegetables, raw, lightly cooked, steamed or juiced.

- Eat fermented foods like sauerkraut to boost the beneficial gut flora & supplement with acidophilus probiotic.

- Onions, Garlic, Ginger, Chives, Coriander, a multitude of fresh herbs and spices. All common garden herbs we deemed as wonderful health promoters and added beautiful flavour enhancement to meals.

- Drink plenty of pure filtered water, one and a half to two litres per day, but not with meals which would neutralise stomach acids inhibiting digestion.

- The importance of chewing food well which releases the amylase digestive enzyme within the mouth which is the first port of digestion. Relaxed mealtimes with no rush.

- Eat small portions of white meat in place of red meat. We ate small amounts of organic chicken and oily fish which is easier for the body to digest (organic or responsibly sourced, no cruel toxic factory farms).

- Drink green tea's and herbal teas which have catechin flavonoid anti-oxidants. Grow herbs and use them for the ultimate fresh tea infusions. Nettle, mint, parsley, sage, thyme, lemon verbena, lavender adding some liquorish root or small amount of local unprocessed organic honey (optional). Just as a note green tea contains caffeine so be mindful not to drink too much, especially at night.

- The juice of lemons diluted with water first thing in the morning to alkalise, re-hydrate and detoxify the body's system, twenty to thirty minutes before food.

- Use a rebounder regularly to move the lymphatic system.

- Use positive affirmations, you can do this Yeaaah!!!

What you do and how you think:

Consider carefully what you do and how you think, a positive mind is a pathway to health and wellbeing.

- Get away from stress and find good wholesome ways of relaxation

- Consider your job and be around uplifting encouraging friends and family.

- Strive to make changes to enable you to enjoy life.

- Have a passion and purpose.

- If practical, pull away from people or situations that drain you. Some people can be termed as psychological vampires that can suck your energy dry.

- Learn how to laugh again

- Getting good aerobic exercise with the feel good highs oxygenating the body well and getting the lymphatic system moving.

- Find a pastime that makes you feel good about yourself.

- Try taking the focus off yourself to help lift other people. Self-focussed people often tend to be unhappy people.

- Do random acts of kindness.

- Forgive and get resentment out of your system

> **Forgiveness is unlocking the door to set someone free and then realizing you were the prisoner!**

- Feel positive, you are going to help your body to mend, it's a great feeling of taking control.

- Absolutely believe in whatever pathway you choose to do. If you believe you can or you believe you can't you will be right on both accounts!

- Spend time in Prayer and ask God, who loves you dearly, for strength, comfort, guidance, wisdom and healing.

Bargaining with life on taste factor

I have outlined the fundamentals of 'what we chose to do' and why we chose to do it, throughout our traumatic experiences. It is for you the reader to make of it what you will and hopefully it will encourage you to do your own research in order to formulate your own healthcare plan of action based on knowledge. Remember we are not giving anyone specific advice and there may very well be more required. Some people do cannabis oil, Gerson protocol, Budwig protocol, Royal Rife – (bio resonance), Essiac tea, Iscador, black salve, etc. etc. We are sharing information as to what we chose to do when my wife was faced with cancer.

I have heard people trying to bargain with their lives with what 'tastes good' or not so good to them, saying:

- "Well I don't like that green leafy stuff and vegi wotsits!"

- "No one is stopping me from having four sugars in my tea!"

- "What do you know, give me a doctor when I am sick, someone who knows what they are talking about!"

- "Oh, but I eat healthily!!!" Followed by glazed blank look.

I have had all of these comments thrown at me and more, even by friends and people I love. Only you can decide to make the conscious decision to change nutritional, lifestyle and thought processes that are not serving you well. To continue or discontinue with the foods that induce or feed cancer and many other chronic diseases is our own choice.

Doctors are there to fix when broken and to treat sickness when it has already developed, or you could say after the horse has bolted. It lies solely in your hands to close the stable door, ideally before the horse has bolted (prevention).

We felt that information was the key to turning things around to stack the odds in Sue's favour, but it also called for 'taking response - ability' and personal action. You are too precious to your family and friends to give up, so take heart and positive action to inspire those around you. YOU CAN DO THIS!

In fact why not say it out loud, right now!

Daily Positive affirmations

- I totally believe I am creating a body environment in which cancer is unable to thrive.

- I totally believe I am wrecking the environment that cancer needs to thrive.

- I totally believe that I am beating this cancer as I speak these words into my beautiful cells.

- I totally believe I am starving this cancer of everything it needs.

- I totally believe that I am building up an incredible immune system to fight the cancer.

- I am creating an amazingly healthy body.

- I totally believe I am oxygenating my body in order that cancer cannot survive.

- I totally believe that I have removed all toxicity from my body and mind.

- I now no longer place toxins into my body and my body is beautifully pure temple.

- I love myself, my life and my family and I am going to be around for them some while longer yet.

- I am loved and I am precious and I will heal.

Say this everyday out loud to yourself, over and over as "the power of the spoken word is mighty indeed in pulling down strongholds". So mark this page and revisit it every day and believe it because it is true.

You are beautiful, you are precious, you are valued and you are loved, so go for it!

Key Factors in Western Disease

Through what I have seen, witnessed and researched over the years, I have great concerns regarding the cancer medical industry. There appears to be a total aversion to common sense in the efficacy of nutrition and the vital role it can play in preventative and who knows maybe even curative powers.

The common sense approach should be the realisation that the correct choice of nutrition can serve to be a vital ally in building up the immune system and greatly contribute to the success or failure in the fight against chronic disease.

PubMed Study: "Cancer is a Preventable Disease that Requires Major Lifestyle Changes" (Published online 2008 Jul 15) The study states that 90 to 95% of cancers are attributed to environmental and lifestyle factors. So surely it is important to address these issues to rectify and to avoid health problems even if people choose to go down the medical treatment route.

When the body is nutritionally deficient and food contains chemical toxicity, we know that this can cause inflammation and auto immune responses, i.e. the immune system attacking self.

I believe without a shadow of doubt that under nourishment of essential vitamins, minerals, enzymes and live foods coupled with our modern agricultural food toxicity and dead processed foods, that these all play key roles in leading to many of today's westernised diseases. Making changes to redress these deficiencies, toxicity and changing the body's internal environment, we firmly believe can and as in my wife's cancer situation has, served to turn things around.

Try to look at cancer from another angle. The cancer, lump or tumour 'is not the cancer'; it is the 'symptom' of the underlying holistic cancer problem. Whilst the cancer industry continues to view the lump or the bump as the cancer and persist in treating the symptoms not the cause, there will be no real cures on the horizon. What we will predominantly see is remissions, treatments, remissions, treatments remissions treatments which continue to amass incredible profits for the corporate pharmaceutical companies.

Cancer Nutrition at its Best?

I visited a dear person to us on a cancer ward recently, where I witnessed a hospital porter taking round a large two tiered trolley packed with chocolate bars, sweets, crisps, fizzy sugary drinks and energy drinks, DEAD FOOD! These foods were certainly not conducive to what I would term as convalescence foods in building up the immune system of very poorly people with cancer. However the cancer patients on the ward were buying products that were highly processed, acidifying, deoxygenating, sugar inducing without any live organisms for pro-life. My friend and I watched and looked knowingly at each other with sadness in our hearts.

I have watched and stood by whilst hospitals gave sugar, starchy foods (sugar forming) processed red meat, old reheated, dried up food, ice cream, apple pie and sugary buns and milk to people that I love when they were being treated with cancer.

This breaks my heart, especially now that I have a greater understanding and the scales have been removed from my eyes. These people (my family) were very poorly which was compounded by the debilitating treatments and yet even further compounded by the type and quality of nutrition they received.

They deserved better, to be treated holistically with immune boosting nutrition to enable them fight and recover, not foods that fed the cancer and created a bodily environment in which cancer thrived. My family were denied this and the consequences were that our hearts broken by the loss of our loved ones!

A Diet for Chemotherapy?

By Chris Woollams of Canceractive, to whom I have the greatest respect.

"One of our readers was having chemotherapy and picked up an NHS booklet at the Royal Marsden on ´A Diet for Chemotherapy´. It covered recommendations on what to eat as a cancer diet when undergoing chemotherapy. And she was horror struck".

"I thought it was some sort of April Fool", she wrote in her letter to us.

Small pictures of a cheeseburger, a milkshake and a sticky bun or cake on every page, with recommendations to drink milky sugary tea, consume cows´ dairy, sugar and fats were commonplace. Is this really a cancer diet for cancer patients? Is this cancer nutrition at its best? A diet to beat cancer"?

"We quizzed the hospital, for whom we have the greatest respect. The reply stated that the sole issue during chemotherapy was to keep up body weight, hence the diet full of calories from fats and sugar". Only recently in a Times review on cancer, an 'expert' reiterated this fat and glucose rich diet, telling cancer patients - ALL cancer patients on chemotherapy that calories were good and they should have lots of cows' dairy and sugary foods to keep their weight up! Yet we are all told regularly in the media that this is a 'junk diet' to be avoided at all costs".

Isn't this processed food, high sugar diet supposed to be massively implicated in the cause of cancer?

On my soap box

Most people seem to be oblivious to the state of the world's agricultural industry today, through short-sighted unsustainable corporate greed. The soil in which we grow our food today is so depleted of essential minerals and nutrients that this in turn causes sick deficient produce. The answer of modern corporate agriculture seems to be that we spray it with toxic pesticides, herbicides, larvicides and fungicides along with the use of synthetic fertilisers and growth stimulating chemicals. Is this the best way to produce food that we hope will sustain us and keep ourselves, our families and our future descendants healthy?

We should also consider the far reaching implications of genetically modified (GM) crops and their effect on wildlife biodiversity, nature and ultimately human health. We as consumers usually turn a blind eye to these things, but my thoughts are that if the bugs and bacteria do not want to eat it then why would we? We perhaps do not realise the full implications of these GM foods and the extent that these unnatural abominations are in our food chain, largely through processed foods.

We are told that GM foods will help to feed the world, when in reality their yields are far inferior to that of naturally produced crops. Try looking into why over one hundred thousand farmers in India have committed suicide due to their failing GM crops and massive debts incurred by having to turn to the corporate seed producer for more expensive patented seeds and chemicals.

For the first couple of years bumper crops and then decimation having to go back to the GM company to buy more high priced seeds and pesticide which financially cripple them. This is serious business and it is not about the goodness and virtue of feeding the world, it is about corporate greed, profits and power.

I would further go on to say, the potential of corporations controlling our very food by patenting seeds and nature. If as a consequence people are poisoned in the process, then the other arm of the pharmaceutical companies will make money off treating your sickness too. How corrupt, how dangerous, how powerful the control of corporations, to own patented rights to nature and the very food we eat. I believe we should fight this corruption at all costs.

Remember the House of Commons has a food procurement policy for our MPs which stipulate that they do not have genetically modified (GM) foods served in the House of Commons. If GM crops are so great then why don't they want to eat it and why is there this stipulation against GM?

Unhealthy oils and fats

Should we be eating synthetic hydrogenated fats and trans-fatty acids (margarines), that our body does not recognise as food and are one molecule away from being plastic? These unnatural fats eventually build up within the cardio vascular system and arterial walls to cause a hardening and contribute to high blood pressure, strokes and cardiovascular problems.

Frying and heating up vegetable cooking oils is widely known to cause carcinogenic toxins to be released into our food, but we do not seem to question their health effect, coz they taste so good!!! Our body is unable to process these unnatural toxic fats so they end up like a plaque coating and clogging up the body causing all sorts of health issues. These harmful fats are found in most processed foods today, but we still keep munching obliviously unaware.

Plastics and Bisphenol A (BPA)

We continue heating and cooking our foods in plastic containers which release toxins such as Biphenyl A. (BPA) into our food. These plastics along with others like PVC mimic the female hormone oestrogen with the abilities to influence cancer growth and the potential to cause genetic hormonal abnormalities, especially in young developing children. These same plastics exuding particularly BPA are being used in many products such as baby's formula bottles, dummies, sterilisation heat units, food containers, plastic bags, condoms, lining of cans, shrink wrap, kettles and many more everyday items. Such products are known to be carcinogenic, and hormone mimicking and hormone disrupters especially when heated or used over a continual period of time enabling the toxins slow but consistent release.

BPA is an organic compound and is used to make flexible plastics and epoxy resins. BPA has been used commercially since 1957 and around 3.6 million tonnes (8 billion pounds) of BPA are used within manufacturing processes every year. Plastics with BPA are normally clear and durable, which makes it a very popular and common choice for consumer goods like baby bottles and water bottles, sports equipment, and CDs and DVDs. Additionally it is used for industrial purposes, like lining water pipes and epoxy resins used as coatings on the inside of many food and beverage cans.

BPA is able to leach out of the plasticised products into the food we consume. Don't let us forget the innocent looking teabags that contain plastic, either 100% polypropylene or 20% epoxy plasticized paper to prevent the bag from tearing as normal paper would do when in contact with water.

BPA exhibits hormone-like properties which mimic oestrogen which raises concern about its suitability in consumer products and food containers. Several governments have questioned its safety in recent years, which prompted some retailers to withdraw polycarbonate products. A published report in 2010 from the United States Food and Drug Administration (FDA) warned of possible hazards to foetuses, infants, and young children.

In September 2010, Canada became the first country to declare BPA a toxic substance. The European Union, Canada, and recently the United States have now banned BPA use in baby's bottles. With our abundant plastic waste and chemical contaminations of waterways we are now seeing male fish turning female. BPA is also termed as a xenoestrogen which is a synthetic imitator of the female hormone oestrogen and is known to be an endocrine system hormone disrupter.

Meat

Western cultures eat large amounts of meat and in particular red meat which depletes our body of massive amounts of energy and digestive enzyme resources in order to break it down for the body to absorb. Red meats particularly take a prolonged time to go through the bowels, this prolonged processing allows the meat to putrefy in the bowels creating a re-absorption of putrefying toxins into the body. I understand that many diseases start to develop from within the bowels.

> "Please test your servants for ten days; Give us nothing but vegetables to eat and water to drink".
>
> Daniel, Chapter 1, Verse 16.

Meat consumption is also highly acidifying and should be eaten in moderation i.e. smaller palm of the hand sized portions and eaten less frequently. Livestock are also routinely treated with antibiotics, steroids and growth stimulating hormones. We also need to be conscious of the conditions of the livestock and stresses they have endured and what they have been fed. All of these factors come together in determining whether the meat is from a healthy or sick animal and what toxins they may transfer to us through into the food chain.

Hydration

Our water is mineral deficient contaminated with hormones like oestrogens, sodium fluoride (main constituent of rat poison) toxic Chlorine additive. We tend not to drink enough 'pure water' to regularly flush out the body to allow efficient detoxification. We do however fill our bodies with caffeinated drinks which are acidifying and are known diuretics which serve to take more fluid out of the body to process the caffeine than they do to hydrate the body. End result, further dehydration of the already dehydrated body.

Without a fully hydrated body our functions and detoxifying capabilities are severely compromised. We also may become more prone to the loss of synovial fluid from joints which will become stiff, painful and inflamed as in rheumatoid arthritis. Drinking a litre and a half to two litres of pure water is vitally important to our overall health.

Processed foods the norm

Culturally we eat unnatural processed, preserved, artificial fatty foods and reconstituted foods. These foods are also regularly fed to our children in schools from an early age and we expect no repercussions, but it tastes good people say.

The processing of milk and dairy is a real eye opener to anyone who cares to look beyond the cute picture of the cow on the plastic carton. As discussed earlier; the milk of today is not the same milk that I remember when I was growing up as a child.

No one is saying that you are not able to have drinks you like or even that cream bun, but if this is frequent then just bear in mind that you may have to deal with the consequences of your choices sooner or later. It is not any of my business or my intention to look down on anyone's choices in food and lifestyle. If the person

We aimed for 80% alkali forming foods and 20% acid forming for a good balance.

consumes excessive acidifying foods, large quantities of meat, processed foods, fatty foods, preserved and reconstituted foods, processed sugars and artificial sweeteners, M.S.G. along with vitamin and mineral depleted chemical ladened fruits and vegetables then this will place a great strain on the body and its ability to fight infection and disease. The stomach feels full and satisfied, but the body is left crying out in a very vulnerable and nutritionally depleted state, a full stomach, but starving to death on a cellular level.

Please do not stand in the highway saying I do not believe in cars and trucks. The reality is that whatever your belief you will soon be educated to the consequences of your actions and be hit with reality.

The Cause for Cancer

There is so much evidence that cancer is largely a metabolic issue that it beggars belief how it can be ignored to this extent by the medical fraternity. Just as Scabies, Rickets and pellagra were proved to be the lack of vitamins C, D and B3. It is interesting to note that the medical profession initially refuted these facts too and pilloried the scientists behind these findings until they could deny it no longer in the face of the overwhelming evidence. The evidence is now building up for cancer as well.

CANCER "Everyone should know that the 'war on cancer' is largely a fraud."

Dr. Linus Pauling, the only person ever to win two solo Nobel Prizes.

I think that in years to come people will look back on these days of current cancer treatments as being very dark days of ignorance and mass deception for corporate power and profit. I find it quite incredible that when the medical establishment's studies say that up to 90-95% percent of cancers may be attributed to environmental factors including poor nutrition/lifestyle, that they pursue 'early diagnosis' and place great emphasis on this rather than educating people in what constitutes preventative and healthy nutrition.

Bare these figures in mind of 90-95% never getting cancer in the first place against the figures of the chemotherapy contribution to the five year survival rates of 2.1% USA and 2.3% Australia. You could in effect slash billions off our financially crippled NHS and save so much pain and suffering through educating our children from an early age in what constitutes a healthy lifestyle and healthy nutrition. However, it may be that there is just too much money at stake for the processed food corporations who sing the public a beautiful pied piper song of what their products will do for us.

The taste, the texture, the convenience, the price, the shelf life, the feel good factor of satiation and flavour enhancing chemicals. The morishness, the addictiveness!!! The reality is however somewhat different from the advertisement hype of the manufacturers when you become obese, sick, arthritic, heart problems, eczema, diabetes, cancer etc. etc.

> "Intellectually bankrupt, fiscally wasteful and therapeutically useless", said Dr. James Watson, (Nobel Laureate) when asked about cancer research and the National Cancer Program.

This is where the pharmaceutical corporations step up and come in on the scene making billions in medications, drugs and treatments from the consequences of their ugly twin sister the processed food industry.

To me, spending multiple millions in early diagnosis of cancer without the education of well documented factors implicated in causing cancer seems to be outrageous and morally corrupt. The system pays lip service to the "eat your five a day" mantra but in my mind this is not going far enough in reconnecting people with the importance of properly constituted nutrition in alleviating many chronic diseases. When questioning oncologists they seem to tell us that there is no real reason for cancer we don't really know why it happens apart from smoking and the sun.

For the sceptic or person who looks outside the box, I could understand them posing the following question: is this mass campaign for early diagnosis just a recruitment drive for the multibillion per year cancer business steered by the pharmaceutical companies?

Oncologists can keep cutting out the cancer, poisoning and burning the tumours along with poisoning the rest of the body's good cells, but unless they are prepared to address the fundamental reasons the person succumbed to the cancer in the first place, then the cancer can and more often

> The famous French writer 'Voltaire, said that the art of medicine consists of amusing the patient while nature cured the disease.

than not does keep on coming back. But perhaps you shouldn't worry too much because you are in good hands as they will treat you, treat you, treat you, and treat you again. All of this whilst ignoring known nutritional and lifestyle factors!

Imagine, if you came home to a flood in the kitchen and the taps were fully on, water flooding over the sink, which would you go for first, the mop or the taps? I hope that no one said the mop! Any person in their right mind would of course go for the source of the problem.

If you believe that the tumour is the cancer and simply remove it or poison it, then you are just mopping up instead of dealing with the underlying source of the problem (turning off the taps). You would in effect be trying to dry yourself off whilst still in the shower. It is ridiculous to believe that you can ever cure a predominantly 'metabolic or toxicity' problem with drugs, but you can treat it, and treat it and treat it. No drug ever cured scurvy, pellagra or rickets, these were cured with good wholesome fresh food and nutrition (vitamin deficiencies).

> **"Correctly Prescribed Drugs Take Heavy Toll**
>
> **Millions Are Affected By Toxic Reactions"**
>
> "More than two million Americans become seriously ill every year because of toxic reactions to 'correctly prescribed' medicines taken properly, and 106,000 die from those reactions, a new study concludes. That surprisingly high number makes drug side effects at least the sixth, and perhaps even the fourth, most common cause of death in this country".
>
> **The Washington Post**
>
> Wednesday, 15th April 1998

There has been a massive amount of research done into nutrition and cancer but this appears to have been largely ignored by the allopathic medical establishment. If you ask any GP about nutrition it's a bit like going into a Chinese restaurant and asking for a chicken Rogan

Josh, it simply is not on the menu, they do not know how to make it and you're not going to get it.

It is a fact that GP's receive little or no training in nutrition, they are however highly trained in medicine to prescribe pharmaceutical medication and drugs only!

There are eighteen different cultures living in the world 'today' that amazingly do not have cancer, sugar diabetes, cardio vascular disease or any other western diseases for that matter.

The Hunzakut tribe of the Himalayas, The Abkasions of Russia, Okinawans in Japan, Titicaca Indians from Peru. This is not widely publicized but these cultures do exist and they regularly live in excess of one hundred years of age in extremely good health. Check this out for your selves in a book called 'The Blue Zones' by Dan Buettner. If this does not ring any alarm bells for people I don't know what will. But hang on a minute, there are no rocket scientists living in these areas to work out the cellular or genetic actions of the food they eat in relation to the bodies processes etc. There are no cancer specialists, no dentists because they are living life the way nature intended.

If these facts are true, (and you need to satisfy yourselves that they are) then it suggests that there is something fundamentally wrong with the way westernised cultures live and what we consume. I will leave you to reach your own conclusions as to the ethics of the cancer industry and their symbiotic relationship with the pharmaceutical companies and regulatory authorities.

I do not believe in a silver bullet, nor any snake oil cure for that matter, because clearly it is a whole lifestyle within westernised culture that is causing us to fall like flies to cancer and many other chronic and not so chronic illnesses. Some of these issues may be beyond our control, but food and nutrition rank high up in the equation of our poor health in the west and this we do have in our power to address which is called 'epigenetics'.

I must make it absolutely clear that I hold in high esteem many aspects of modern medicine and our GP's and doctors, such as A&E trauma and pain management, short term life saving sensible use of antibiotics etc. I also in no way demonise doctors working in the cancer industry as they are certainly very intelligent highly trained people, into a regime that they are moulded into and no doubt they believe in with best intentions.

These doctors are not allowed to step outside of their remit of medication, radiation and surgery otherwise they will lose their jobs and are struck off. My opinion is that they are like boxers going into the ring fighting with one arm tied behind their back. All the doctors are trained in and know is what has been funded and institutionalised by the pharmaceutical companies who are multi billion pound a year corporate giants, with their shareholders to satisfy.

It may be difficult to comprehend the massive implications of this, but we should try to think a little outside of the box and not just bury our heads in the sand like an ostrich hoping that the dangerous predator will go away. Please don't throw yourself off of a ten story building saying I don't believe in gravity. Reality has a tendency to catch up with you despite what your belief is.

I hope that this book has served to answer some of the questions from the sceptic's amongst you. I know through experience that some people, perhaps with good reason would prefer not to know these things as it is often too painful to contemplate. Such a betrayal of trust by the very institutions that we entrust our lives and those of our loved ones is hard to take in. I too have lost people that I love dearly to cancer. At the time things occurred with orthodox treatment that were so blatantly out of order I do not know how I could have stood by and watched it taking place. That is another story though.

It is horrific to think that our medical Universities and teaching institutions are founded and under girded to this day by the pharmaceutical companies, originating from the financial elitists John D Rockefeller, Andrew Carnegie and JP Morgan who invested heavily into newly birthing allopathic medicine in the early 1900s.

When giving all of this funding they made stipulations that if they were going to invest in new hospital buildings, equipment, drugs etc. as a condition, would it be possible for us to have our people to sit on the board of directors to ensure that our money is being spent wisely. This was the birth of the mighty allopathic health system that controlled all the learning within the universities and health educational establishments through the pharmaceutical companies influence.

If our food hygiene inspectors were funded by the restaurant owners we might raise an eyebrow as to their compromised impartiality. Well, this is exactly what we allow to happen with the massive multi billion pound pharmaceutical giants with corporate agendas and their shareholders to satisfy. Everything that our doctors, G.P's surgeons, nurses are trained in has been put in place by these financial corporations and financial elitists with the prime aim being power and to make massive profits. Do you really think it is about health? Show me a healthy person who is on long term pharmaceutical medications.

The Food and Drug Administration (FDA) is also part of this symbiotic relationship and do little to promote nutrition, vitamins or life giving water consumption. In fact quite to the contrary the FDA is anti-herbs, vitamins and natural ways to deal with the many western ailments.

The FDA has recently succeeded in banning use of intravenous vitamin C, as they say it might be dangerous. All of this concern over natural substances but no reservations about genetically altering foods without thorough testing of the full implications. However, once GMO's are out there in nature, there is no retraction and no going back. How forward

> "Genetic engineering has never been about saving the world, it's about controlling the world".
>
> Vandana Shiva

thinking and how health and safety conscious is this to the biodiversity of wildlife and ultimately to human health?

Vitamin C oxygenates the blood and is known to be a serious cancer fighting treatment (ref; Nobel Prize winner Linus Pauling). On the other side of the coin, the FDA endorse the use of highly toxic chemotherapy and radiotherapy both of which have a damning track record of killing and seriously damaging literally millions of people over the years even before they have chance to die from the cancer.

Peer Reviewed Cancer Study

A damning revelation to the ineffectiveness, toxicity and excessive cost of Chemotherapy.

The Royal College of Radiologists conducted their 'peer reviewed study' published by Elsevier Ltd. in 2004,
(Clinical Oncology 16:549e560 doi:10.1016/j.clon.2004.06.007).

"The Contribution of Cytotoxic Chemotherapy to Five Year Survival in Adult Malignancies". *(cytotoxic means poisonous or toxic to cells.)*

The aims of the study state the following:
"The debate on the funding and availability of cytotoxic drugs raises questions about the contribution of curative or adjuvant cytotoxic chemotherapy to survival in adult cancer patients".

The results of the review state:
"The overall contribution of curative and adjuvant cytotoxic chemotherapy to 5-year survival in adults was estimated to be 2.3% in Australia and 2.1% in the USA".

The conclusion of the study states:
"As the 5-year relative survival rate for cancer in Australia is now over 60%, it is clear that cytotoxic chemotherapy only makes a minor contribution to cancer survival. To justify the continued funding and availability of drugs used in cytotoxic chemotherapy, a rigorous evaluation of the cost-effectiveness and impact on quality of life is urgently required. Morgan, G. et al. (2004). Clinical Oncology 16, 549e560 _ 2004 The Royal College of Radiologists. Published by Elsevier Ltd".

The 2004 peer reviewed study speaks for itself, a near ninety eight percent ineffectiveness in cytotoxic chemotherapies contribution to the five year survival in adult malignancies. All we need to do is look around and ask ourselves if the claims of the cancer industry are true, which constantly appear in the media, the claims that we are winning the war on cancer. If winning the war on cancer means that one in two people are getting cancer, (CRUK) then what losing the battle would be like?

This constant and relentless media flow is being funnelled into the minds of the public as mind persuasive propaganda articles, using words like 'new treatment on the horizon', pioneering research, paving the way, 'further down the line' , 'in a few years', 'we hope to', 'might', 'maybe'.

There words always appear to be carefully chosen to be non-committal and usually followed by a request for more of your money and together 'we will beat this disease'. The truth is that we are still using three core treatments in orthodox cancer treatment which have remained unchanged for the last seventy to one hundred years;

1. Radiotherapy, (first used circa 1895*)

2. Chemotherapy (first used circa 1940 originating from a chemical warfare 'nerve/mustard gas' designed and used to kill people)

3. Surgery (in some situations a viable necessity, in others a butchery service when other natural options seem to be ignorantly swept aside).

Imagine, literally hundreds of billions of pounds raised worldwide for cancer research over the decades. I cannot help but pose the question as to why we are still using predominantly the same highly toxic, highly invasive cancer treatments that cause cancer in themselves. The equipment may have shinier dials, digits, bells and lights on, but fundamentally they remain the same toxic sledgehammers.

Around two million people in America are diagnosed with cancer each year and around three hundred and fifty thousand within the UK. One in two will get the devastating news of a cancer diagnosis at some time in their lives. This is the flip of a coin.

With all the incredible technological advances over the past half-century and orthodox medicine is no closer to finding a "cancer cure," while cancer has grown into a worldwide epidemic of incredible proportions. The statistics are as follows and pretty much speak for themselves:

- In the early 1900's approximately one in thirty people developed cancer
- In the 1940s, approximately one in sixteen people developed cancer
- In the 1970s, one in ten
- Today, one in two will get cancer according to Cancer Research UK (CRUK).

We are forever being told that we are winning the war on cancer, but are we really?

Oncologists are often promoting to cancer patients new promising trials which the lucky person could be placed on, but patients must act quickly. It is akin to used car salesman techniques pressurising Come on come on buy it NOW as there is a limited time for the deal, this a special one chance offer and the pressure mounts to make the decision quickly.

The costs of these new trials are so incredibly expensive that patients believe they are so lucky to be chosen for these pioneering treatments. It breaks my heart when I continue to hear cancer patients saying how lucky they are for

> Our food has changed more in the last fifty years than in the last ten thousand years.
>
> Work out the correlation with the explosion of today's prevalent common western diseases.

this opportunity. We then hear later more often than not that did not make it and they passed away.

We actually have a diet for cancer booklet from an eminent hospital in England that unashamedly states:

"Do not bulk up on fruits and vegetables".

Patients are then encouraged to eat sugar and fats, cakes, buns, dairy, burgers and meat as if these bore no consequence.

Fizzy sugary drinks, chocolate bars sweets and potato crisp dispensers on virtually every oncology ward and throughout hospitals. Hospital cafés with cakes, pies, puddings, processed meat, chips with no sight of fresh green herbs, vegetables, juices etc.

By 8 years old a child in USA has consumed more sugar than the average person did in their entire lifetime just a century ago

This makes me so angry with a passion, so much so that we want to shout our message from the roof tops to those with an ear to hear who wish to listen.

We firmly believe that Cancer does not just happen and that there are definite reasons which the medical establishment seem to walk around this massive elephant in the living room to keep in favour of highly profitable toxic pharmaceutical drugs and treatments.

Genetically Flawed

Flaw in the theory of Genetics or family predispositions

When you see an obese lady walking along the road holding hands with her young children, one on each side and you notice that both children are on the large size, do you think that the children inherited the obesity gene? Is it not more logical to reason that as a family they most likely eat the same unhealthy foods, have similar inactive lifestyles? Are we not the sum total of what we focus on, consume and mentally absorb?

If all the family were to adopt a healthier more natural diet along with appropriate exercise there would be a massive likelihood that their so called genetic disorder would be overridden by epigenetics and they would become slimmer and healthier.

This same concept I would argue would run true for many westernised chronic disease including cancer when we are told that cancer is in our genes. Whilst there may be predispositions (5-10%) to cancer my logic would tell me that this is far over ridden by epigenetics of lifestyle and nutritional factors.

Knowledge the Key to Empowerment

Anyone who is considering undertaking chemotherapy or radiotherapy would do well to gain as much knowledge as they can to make informed decisions. You are entitled to demand from the oncologist a copy of the MSDS sheets (Material Safety Data Sheets) and to review the information at hand with a supporting friend or family member. Try to rationalise and come to terms with all the implications and effects of what you are agreeing to be treated with.

Doctors will not normally offer the MSDS to patients but it is your right to have this information. Surprisingly the very same radiotherapy and chemotherapy 'cure' has the unfortunate

> My People Perish Through Lack of Knowledge
>
> Hosea Ch 4. Vs 6. KJV

side effect of being carcinogenic (cancer causing), and obliterating the immune system, which is often one of the very reasons why the patient succumbed to cancer in the first place.

Material safety data sheets can sometimes appear to speak in a different type of language (i.e. medical spiel) as who would know what a category one carcinogen means? Well it means 'known to cause cancer in humans' and Category two carcinogen meaning 'thought to cause cancer in humans'. How are you ultimately going to create a healthy body using treatments that cause hair, nails and teeth to fall out and that make you vomit, that burn you with radiation and are mutagenic and oh by the way, I will mention it again, cause cancer?

Even if you choose to go down the pathway of conventional orthodox treatment, it is still vitally important to pack your body full of the best nutrition you can in order to build up your immune system which is going to be in for a stormy ride from conventional chemotherapy and radiotherapy. I read that by fasting for three days prior to chemotherapy that this enhances the protection to normal cells whilst targeting the cancer cells.

If all this information does is to make you think and then research for yourself then at least you will be making an informed decision, whichever pathway you decide is right for you.

The basic principle of building up the body's immune system with the finest nutrition and implementing positive lifestyle strategies surely has to be common sense, whether going through cancer or not. Consuming fresh nutritious foods, free from processing and toxicity, adequate sleep, reduced stress, well hydrated body, adequate sunlight, to be loved and to be happy are all things that help us to maintain our overall health and wellbeing.

The information contained in this book should not be seen as condemning anyone for their food and lifestyle choices, but an education into the natural empowering protocols which my wife and I chose to do when faced with cancer.

Speaking out that people may be harming themselves through their daily food choices or lifestyle can and often does cause great offence, but this is far from my intention. This book should be seen as information to enable people to make up their own minds as to its credibility. Many processed foods are designed to be addictive (MSG, Aspartame, Sugar HFCS), so you can be forgiven in finding it difficult to make changes. I still struggle myself with eating things that I am aware are not the best for me, but even implementing small changes in the right direction and building on this are all steps forward in a healthier direction.

People often tell me "well I eat healthily, I read all the labels"! I listen respectfully to what they say, but often they do not have any foundation to base their claim, as to what constitutes a healthy diet. Fresh produce is not grown with a label on it with long chemical words you cannot pronounce let alone spell! Even the so called fresh produce grown by mass corporate agriculture is grown in nutritionally depleted soils and chemically sprayed, so does this constitute eating healthy?

Society seems to have gotten lost and confused somewhere along the way. We would prefer to buy that big house or car or beautiful clothes rather than invest in the best organic super foods to keep ourselves and our family in great health. I have listened enough to the manipulative advertising of corporate processed food manufacturers that seduces our nation and our children to their own profitable ends.

Making important changes to lifestyle habits can serve to stack the odds in the cancer sufferer's favour. You would definitely not pour petrol on the bonfire to put it out would you? Then with the same concept, do not provide cancer with the ideal environmental conditions and the fuel that it needs to thrive.

The Cruise Ship Analogy

By Nicola Cororan

My analogy of a cancer diagnosis is one of having lived my entire life on a cruise liner. I never had to think about steering this ship, or where I was going. I gorged on the buffet laid out before me, without consciousness. It was easy, but unsatisfying.

On diagnosis I felt that I had been cast out of the liner into a small row boat. Attached to the rest of society by a flimsy rope, life became a struggle to keep up. I felt isolated. Friends and family, still aboard the liner, waved at me eating cake, drinking wine, cheering me on. And I looked up longingly, misguidedly thinking that all I wanted was to get back onto that ship.

Over time I started to look around me, to see the beauty of life inside my boat, the responsibility that I now embraced, and the madness of life on the liner. I began to steer my little boat, and wish that others (cancer free of course) could join me in the beauty of my adventure.

I cut the rope.

Sometimes the storms down here are rough, but they are never less than exciting. I feel connected to the waves, vibrant and alive. I am constantly learning how to navigate this journey.

And when I look closely, I see a community of little boats, an armada. I am not alone. I never was. I was just in the wrong boat.

Squirrels and Robins

The robin was a very special fellow to my father as his feathery friend often used to hang around Dads allotment for worms etc. The robin used to get so close and often used to stand on dads fork or spade handle.

Dad was feeling really low the night before his brain tumour operation. This was unusual for him as he was always very positive throughout his cancer. My father had a tremendous faith in God which I suppose gave him a great deal of reassurance. My sisters and I tried to encourage Dad to go out into the hospital gardens and we eventually managed to persuade him.

As we approached a large tree in the garden, we saw four squirrels chasing around the ground. They proceeded to run up into the tree in quite a frenzy. This was so lovely to see, but then they started to drop nuts off the tree, two hitting my sister. We laughed so much which lifted our spirits including my dad's.

We then sat on the park bench about six feet away from a bush. A little robin came and rested in the bush directly in front of us. He was so beautiful and unafraid and just stayed there for a good while. This was a very special time that I will never forget because the sombre mood was beautifully lifted in this very difficult time.

Mr Robin often came to visit my dad when he was in the Hospice and chirped up the atmosphere just at the right time we needed him. This is why the robin is a very special fellow to us.

There was one other wonderful robin experience with Sue on the night of being told she had cancer. The Doctor had prescribed her Tamazepam sleeping tablets because he said that you are going to need them. On that evening Sue couldn't sleep and was considering taking the tablets. At about 2am on the January morning she heard a little tweeting of what she believed to be a robin and this gave her great comfort and she calmly fell to sleep.

Final Words

I hope that this information will serve to inspire and encourage you to do your own research and to take some positive steps forward in your health and wellbeing. Discern your information, where does it come from, who is saying it, why are they saying it, what would happen to that person if they did not say what they were saying and what's in it for them.

Learn the boundaries and limitations of what doctors are allowed or not allowed to tell people. There are many good doctors that recognise the importance of nutrition and there are many that tell you that you may as well suck on boiled sugary sweets or have burger meals all day because food bares no relevance to cancer. Hopefully you are now in a better position to decide for yourself what the right way is for you.

We are planning to hold meetings for educational and support purposes around the UK, so please get in touch if you would like to attend our next event or organise an event for us to give a presentation. We are here to support and encourage, by teaching, explaining and clarifying the concepts of 'what we chose to do' when my wife was faced with cancer.

Please do share this information and please support us by recommending our book to others who you believe may benefit from the information it contains.

Thank you to all those who took the time to pray for Sue throughout this dark time as God certainly moved in wonderful ways, giving strength, comfort and ultimately total healing to her.

Please never forget the power of prayer, even if you do not know God, or are unsure, He knows you and loves you very much. It is never too late to call out to Him and ask for Him to come into your heart and life.

The prevalence of western disease is a consequence of man's greed, manipulation and power which goes hand in hand with our free will to do things our way with God on the outside of our lives. What a corrupt state we find our world in!

I certainly do not pretend to have all the answers, but if you would like to discuss any of the above information and our experience further, then please do not hesitate to get in touch.

May God bless you and bring comfort, healing and health into your life in Jesus name.

Our prayers are with you on your healing journey

Robert and Sue Olifent xx

Healing Testimonies

Active Cancer Therapy Support (ACTS) put on monthly seminars where we simply share Sue's testimony of the natural healing principles that we chose to do when faced with a hopeless situation. We provide support through the sharing of knowledge to people going through cancer or anyone who is caring for someone going through cancer. Our seminars are also open to people who are in realisation of the epidemic statistics of one person in two who will get cancer and want to find out more on the preventative measures to take.

As always, we never give specific advice, all we do is to share information for people to do their own research and make informed decisions concerning their own healthcare options. We are now receiving feedback from many people who by following similar natural principles no longer have signs of physiological activity of cancer.

This is the story of John Mackenzie who we were introduced to through Facebook. John was given no hope, as his kidney cancer had metastasised to his lungs with fifteen tumours in all. Emma, Johns partner, believed totally in the body's natural capacity to heal and she threw everything into stacking the odds in John's favour. John witnessed his lung tumours reducing in size to just scar tissue and it has now been confirmed that there is no physiological activity of the cancer. We were privileged to have John and Emma share their personal testimony at our 'Wake Up to Health' seminar in July 2015, where they inspired so many people.

John Mackenzie Cancer healing testimony

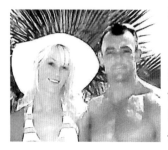

By Emma Collins 05 August 2015

In October 2013 John was diagnosed with kidney cancer and on the 5th December he had surgery to remove the kidney with no further treatment. It was also noted that some nodules were apparent on John's lung, but this was suspected to be inflammation at this time. After discussing dietary health with John, we went on an alkaline diet and included Apricot Kernels (Vitamin B17) just as a precaution and at his next check-up the nodules on his lungs were no longer present.

On John's second check-up In May 2014 we were given the all clear, but the doctors suggested that they would like to keep an eye on him regarding the nodules they had seen previously. In September 2014 John underwent a biopsy of the urethra due to experiencing discomfort, but results again came back as inflammation.

John went back to a normal diet and lifestyle, of which I had serious concerns about, as I wanted him to stay as alkaline as possible to prevent any possible chance of cancer reoccurrence. I do not think at this time that John was fully on board with the dietary regime and its importance; I was of a different opinion though.

The biggest blow of all came in November 2014 when the check-up showed that the nodules on John's lungs had grown and the original kidney cancer had metastasized to the lungs. We were devastated, but I was adamant with John that we needed to go back on the alkaline diet, supplements and apricot kernels, etc. We went away and enjoyed our Christmas and New Year whilst we awaited an appointment following the oncologist's multidisciplinary team meeting (MDT).

In January 2015 we were again informed that the nodules were lung cancer and that it was very aggressive. The doctor explained that it was terminal, but they may be able to prolong John's life with biological therapy. I begged John not to go down the medical route, but he was scared and wanted to do both the diet and their therapy. The medical professionals were not pleased with my views and said that I must be careful and advise them of everything that John was doing so that it did not react with their treatments.

They scheduled another scan for four weeks' time to see how fast the cancer was growing, so that gave me four weeks to prove to John that he didn't need biological therapy. The medical professionals were not in agreement with my strong belief in natural principles of healing and I felt that the doctors were very rude in their attitude to me. The doctor told me that it was up to John what he wanted to do, not me! I left the hospital telling them that they were in for a shock in four weeks' time as I just knew what I was doing was the right thing to do and so our journey began!

I heard about a couple from Nottingham that healed the wife's terminal liver cancer using natural principles and I made contact on Facebook. Sue was so moved by our situation that she sent us their book free of charge. Susan & Robert Olifent had dedicated their lives to helping others by setting up a cancer support group 'Active Cancer Therapy Support' (ACTS). They put on seminars, sharing their testimony to help and inspire others going through cancer. We spoke to them on the phone which instilled hope into John but understandably John was scared.

We decided to attend one of their seminars in Nottingham. At the seminar we arrived slightly late and we entered into a packed room with standing room only. John knocked the projector and all the paper on the floor, that sure got us noticed but we soon settled in and listened.

Much of what was being said we were actually doing which gave reassurance to John that we were on the right track. I remember actually willing John to listen to Robert and all that he was speaking about. Then came the magic John really needed to hear, Bernie Walsh bless her heart, gave her account of what she did to beat her lung cancer, which immediately got Johns attention. John listened intently to her amazing story of how she beat lung cancer through implementing natural principles learned through attending ACTS seminars. WOW! This was a turning point for John as he actually started to believe. I was so glad we went to the ACTS seminar and so grateful to Bernie for her inspiration.

The day arrived to go for the scan after four weeks of intense dietary, lifestyle and detoxification protocols. We were then called a week later for the scan results. The results were that the thirteen tiny tumours surrounding the two main tumours had gone completely. The 15mm one was now 5mm and the 22mm had shrunk dramatically.

In just four weeks we had made a massive impact and we were so overjoyed. John felt so confident that he had no intention of going ahead with the biological therapy. The doctors suggested that we come back in four months for a further check-up. I simply couldn't wait four months, so after two months I arranged for John to go for a thermography scan, which showed no cancer activity, which was music to our ears.

John kept his medical appointment for the scan in June 2015 as he was keen to show the doctors what we had achieved. The results of the medical scan were two tiny 0.3/4mm blips that the doctor said could be just scar tissue and guess what guys? It was the very same oncologist we had right at the start. I did get to say "do you remember me and what I was doing?" her reply... "yes I do", my reply " I told you, you were in for a shock didn't I?

So if we can do this, then there is hope for everyone!!! The foundations of what we did were based on knowledge, positivity, determination and belief, but also having a wonderful community of lovely new friends to help and encourage us along the way whom we cannot thank enough.

Robert and Susan are a God send and they will always be in my heart. I hope to write my own book someday which will be called 'MY PROMISE' so please look out for this.

I wish much love, good health and a happy life to each and every one of you. Never stop believing as all things are possible when you put your mind to it; John, and Sue are living proof of this.
Emma Collins xxxxxx

References

Books
Cancer Why Were Still Dying to Know the Truth, Philip Day
Great News on Cancer in the 21st Century, Steve Ransom
World Without Cancer, G Edward Griffin
Your life in Your Hands, Professor Jane Plant,
The Gerson Therapy,
Health Wars, Philip Day
Plague Pestilence and the pursuit of Power, Philip Day,
The Cancer business, Pat Ratigan
Dismantling Cancer, Francisco Contreras
Cancer, Step Outside the Box, Ty M. Bollinger
Everything You Need to Know to Help You Beat Cancer-Chris Woollams
Toxic Bite, Philip Day
What Doctors Don't Tell You (UK monthly magazine)
What would Jesus eat, Don Colbert M.D.
50 Critical Cancer Answers, Francisco Contreras
Cancer Therapy, Ralph W. Moss PHD
NHS plc, Alyson, M. Pollock
Food For Thought, Philip Day
The Juice Master Diet, Jason Vale
The pH Miracle, Robert Young
The Bible, (Genesis, Leviticus, Daniel)
The Blue Zones, Dan Buettner
Water Cures, Drugs Kill, Dr F Batmanghelidj
Candida Albicans Leon Chaitow,
Your Body's Many Cries For Water, Dr F Batmanghelidj
The Root Of All Disease, Elmer G Heinrich
Simple Changes, Phillip Day
Eat to Outsmart Cancer, Jenny Phillips
Healing Deliciously, Melanie Gamble, Together Against Cancer

Audio Lectures
Dr Leigh Erin Connealy Audio lecture
The Cure for cancer Summit 2013 (26x one hour lectures)
Healing Cancer World Summit 2012, 13 one hour lectures

The Lost Gerson Cancer Tapes (MP3) one hour lectures from fourteen cancer health specialists
Cancer , The Latest Breakthroughs, Philip Day, Audio CD

Website and educational emails
CancerActive, UK website, Chris Woollams
Joseph Mercola website
Natural News, Mike Adams
Renegade Health, Kevin Gianni
The Food Revolution Network, Ocean Robbins
Crazy Sexy Cancer, Kris Carr,

Films/documentaries/lectures (some online)
The Quest For The Cures, Ty Bollinger
Burzynski, the Movie: Cancer Is Serious Business
Healing Cancer from Inside Out, Documentary
Dr. Christine Horner Smarter Strategies for Breast cancer
Science & Politics of Cancer, G Edward Griffin
Foodmatters. Documentary
The Food Revolution, Jamie Oliver
Healthy at 100, Philip Day (live Australian Tour)
Healing Testimonials, Philip Day
Cut Poison Burn, Documentary
Dr Lorraine Day, Cancer Cure Talk,
Run From The Cure The Rick Simpson Story,
Harry Hoxley, When Healing becomes a Crime,
René Caisse, The story of Essiac Tea
Cancer Is Curable Now, Documentary
Bad Medicine, Cancer Cures, DVD Documentary
Cancer, The Forbidden Cures, Documentary
Cancer Dying to have Known, Documentary
The Truth About Our Food, Documentary
Knives over Forks, DVD Documentary
Food Inc. Documentary
Corporations, Documentary
Hungry for Change, Documentary
Eating, The biggest cause of Disease in the US Today
You're Killing My Son, Sally Roberts BBC Documentary
Hungry for Change, Documentary
Drugging our Children, Documentary

Cure All Diseases, Documentary
They Don't Want You to Know, Cancer Documentary
The Quest for the Cures, Documentary, Ty Bollinger
The Truth About Cancer a Global Quest, Ty Bollinger

Medical literature and Institutes
Cancer Research Uk
Journal of the American Medical Association (JAMA)
Department of Radiation Oncology, Sidney Peer reviewed study into
Chemotherapy Clinical Oncology (2004)
MSDS of chemotherapeutic drugs
World Health Organisation
Pubmed, Peer Reviewed Studies

Personal experience
Nottingham City Hospital,
QMC Hospital
Kings Mill Hospital

Natural Health Organisations/Practitioners
Naturopath, Michael Burt ND, Surrey, UK. 07767 034526
Together Against Cancer Charity (Leicester) 0116 246 0195
Yes to Life, Cancer Charity, 0870 163 2990
CancerActive Charity, UK , Chris Woollams
Cancer Options, Nottingham, Patricia Peat 0114 360 8188
Christopher Etheridge PhD. London-Epping-Essex, 07779 414099
Carley Mellors Blair Healing Touch Academy Nottingham 01159 676434
Gerson Institute, Mexico, Charlotte Gerson
Hope4cancer, Tony Jiminez MD, Mexico
Oasis of Hope cancer centre Mexico, Francisco Contreras,
Hoxey Institute, Mexico
Credence, Phillip Day
Burzynski Clinic USA